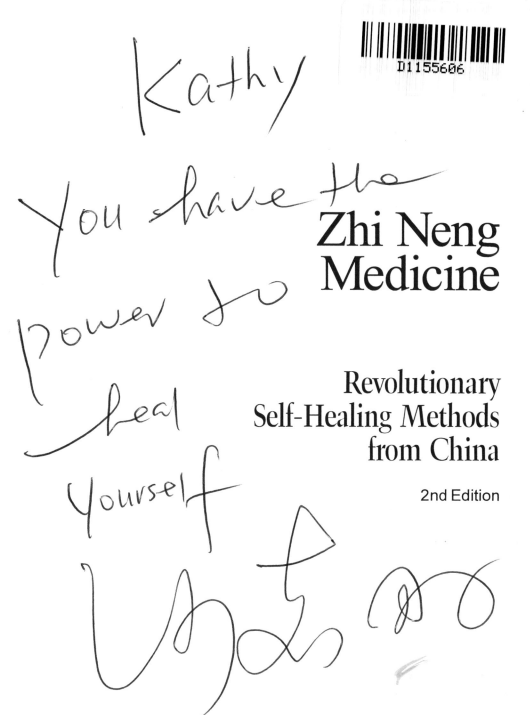

Kathy
You have the
power to
heal
yourself

Zhi Neng Medicine

Revolutionary
Self-Healing Methods
from China

2nd Edition

Zhi Neng Medicine

Revolutionary Self-Healing Methods from China

2nd Edition

Zhi Gang Sha (Xiao Gang Guo)

ZHI NENG PRESS

Vancouver, BC

This book is not intended to replace the services of a health care provider in the diagnosis or treatment of illness or disease.

Any application of the material in this book is at the reader's discretion and is his or her sole responsibility.

Before starting any health or exercise program, the reader should consult a physician.

Physical distress of any kind during or after performing any of the exercises in this book should be carefully monitored as it may indicate a health problem that requires the attention of a health-care professional.

iv **Zhi Neng Medicine**
Revolutionary Self-Healing Methods from China
2nd Edition

Published by Zhi Neng Press
  2nd Edition: May 1997, June 2000, February 2003
  1st Edition: March 1996

For further information:

Zhi Gang Sha LLC
PO Box 470580
San Francisco, CA 94147-0580
Telephone: 1-888-339-6815 (Toll Free)
Website: www.drsha.com

ISBN 0-9680595-2-X

cover design: Heaven
direction: Master Sha
cover illustration: Anand R. Mani
book visuals: Jim Chow

Printed in Vancouver, BC, Canada by Benwell-Atkins.

Preface to the Second Edition

The first printing of this book received a very warm welcome. Thousands of readers, including alternative medicine practitioners and medical professionals, have already incorporated the revolutionary energy development and self-healing techniques of Zhi Neng medicine into their lives for better health.

Many people with cases of chronic pain have improved tremendously with the remarkable self-healing techniques presented in this book. People adopt the methods quickly as they are *simple, effective and easy to learn*. Readers tell us that they love the book for its simplicity, effectiveness and its practicality. Many were excited to find healing techniques that *worked*. Response to the book continues to be very warm.

This second edition of *Zhi Neng Medicine, Revolutionary Self-Healing Methods from China* was produced by May Guey Chew. Given full responsibility to improve upon the first printing, she has produced an even better book. I truly appreciate her total contribution. To Sophia Deer and Steven Wong for helping May – *Thank You!*

"Welcome!" is my greeting to you as you open these pages. *"Welcome to better health! Take Zhi Neng Medicine into your life and let it serve you. Hao! Hao! Hao!"*

Thank you.

Zhi Gang Sha
Vancouver, BC
May 1997

i

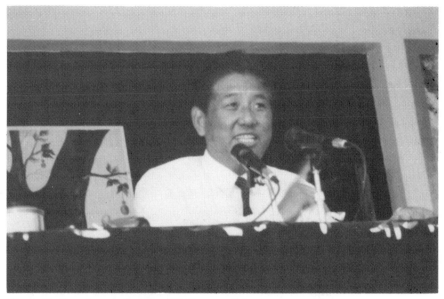

Master Zhi Chen Guo, the founder of Zhi Neng medicine.
photo courtesy of Master Sha

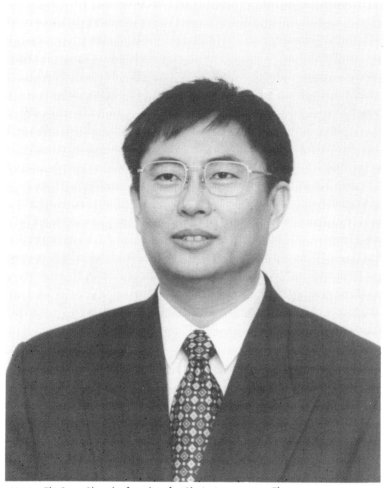

Master Zhi Gang Sha, the founder of *Sha's Acupuncture Therapy.*
photo courtesy of Master Sha

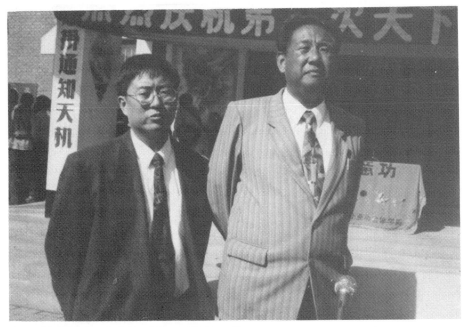

Master Zhi Chen Guo (right) and Master Zhi Gang Sha.
Shijiazhuang, Tian Jing, China, October 1994.
photo courtesy of Master Sha

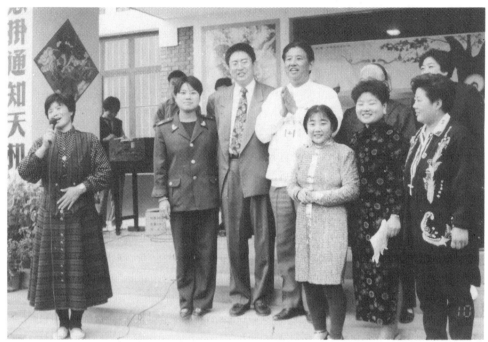

Master Sha with his new family on the day of his adoption, October 1993.
photo courtesy of Master Sha

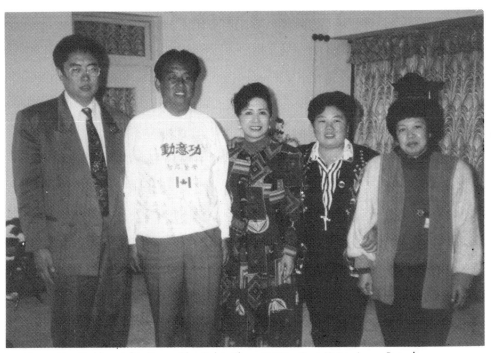

Master Guo (2nd from left), Master Sha, Sylvia Chen, Mei Ling Guo, Miriam Leung Rotenburg.
photo courtesy of Master Sha

v

Dedication

I, Zhi Gang Sha, also known by the adoptive name of Xiao Gang Guo, am the honorary adoptive son and first disciple of Zhi Chen Guo, the founder of Zhi Neng Medicine.

Master Guo has given me the great responsibility of spreading the knowledge, theories, principles and techniques of Zhi Neng medicine to the world.

My life is dedicated to this purpose.

This book comes from my heart and is my gift to the people of the world.

Foreword

On October 19, 1995, I had the utmost privilege of attending, in Ottawa, Master Sha's seminar on Zhi Neng medicine. From the beginning, I was quite impressed by his high level of energy, his passion, his conviction, his clarity and simplicity. With great generosity, he shares his knowledge, practical information, techniques, and he expresses solicitude towards all who suffer. In addition, the fact that Master Sha is qualified in Occidental medicine and in traditional Chinese medicine inspired my confidence, which allowed me to be even more receptive and open to his teachings.

Master Sha is concerned with integrating both the Chinese and western medicines. For him, the human being is fundamentally the same in spite of cultural differences. The human being is one. Only our vision limited by our egotism and our social conditioning gives it an image divided into different parts. In his synthesis, Master Sha allows us to see the human being as a whole, ranging from the cell to the spirit. The priority is given to the spirit, indeed in incarnation, that which connects us to transcendental realities. It is an invitation to leave our limited position of an ant for the one of the eagle, who has a panoramic view which enables him to aim at specific targets according to his needs.

The central element of Zhi Neng medicine is energy. The process of its creation, vibration, diffusion, orientation, equilibrium and existence as a field are studied at different levels... cellular, organ systems, mental states and spiritual dimensions. Zhi Neng medicine's fundamental approach aims at optimizing this energy's functions with special hand positioning, creative visualization, and the making of specific sounds related to the organs.

Master Sha's method meets different schools of thought and certain practices that exist in the Occident. These schools borrow more and more elements of knowledge from the ancient wisdom and healing methods of China, India, etc. Zhi Neng medicine is situated at the crossroads of different civilizations.

Zhi Neng medicine is a simple yet valuable healing method. It combines at the same time and in the same space, physical, psychological and spiritual factors. The method closely reflects its theoretical foundation.

Zhi Neng medicine invites the sufferer to assume more responsibility for his own healing and health development, instead of completely depending on external expertise for his well-being. Many research studies have shown that sick people have more chance of overcoming their stressful illnesses when they believe they have the power to decrease the deleterious effects of bad events on their lives. Other studies have confirmed that ideas and emotions cause the body to secrete chemical substances which can influence our state of health by stimulating or depressing our protective immune system.

I believe that, very soon, some institutions will invite Master Sha to do formal research studies, which will further demonstrate the validity and the effectiveness of Zhi Neng medicine.

I hope that Master Sha's book will be welcomed with open-mindedness, even though our social and cultural conditioning has not taught us how to embody spirituality into our daily and often chaotic lives. Being simple and profound, Master Sha's approach will be largely adopted as a healing and preventive method.

Faudry Pierre-Louis, M.D., F.R.C.P.
Ottawa, 1996

To the Reader

Zhi Neng medicine is a unique combination of traditional Chinese medicine, western medicine, Qi Gong, and the extraordinary functioning of the senses. It is a completely new medical philosophy developed by Grand Master Zhi Chen Guo while in the Qi Gong state. (The Qi Gong state is a level of communication with spiritual masters and the universe.)

In this book, Master Zhi Gang Sha, the first disciple of Master Guo, uses very plain language to explain the principles, theories and techniques of Zhi Neng medicine in the hopes that ordinary people will start taking care of their own health and the health of their friends and relatives. People without extensive medical knowledge can do this just by reading this book.

According to my understanding, Zhi Neng medicine is based on three fundamentals. The first two are Master Guo's Cell Theory and his theories of Field and Energy. The third is the intimate connection of the principles of field and energy to traditional Chinese medicine, Yin/Yang Theory, Five Elements Theory, Tao and Te.

The cell theory in Zhi Neng medicine includes not only the modern biological and medical definitions of the cell, but also the influence of the cell's mechanical vibration and movement. This larger concept of the cell explains what produces the characteristic fields of the cells and the energy in their fields. The state of the body's fields and the energy in them are reflected in the physical condition of the body, whether it be healthy or sick. Zhi Neng medicine also proclaims that cells can be developed. Their resultant motions and energies are related to the messages they transmit.

The field theory of Zhi Neng medicine categorizes fields into universal fields and human-body fields. Universal fields consists of all the known physical fields such as magnetic, electrical, and gravitational fields, including the characteristic fields of traditional Chinese medicine such as wind, cold, dryness, dampness, heat and fire. The human-body fields consist of material fields and fields of the mind. The material fields are the foundations of the fields of the mind, but the latter controls and dominates the former. When the universal fields and the human-body fields combine into one entity, they form the unification of heaven and man as it is known in Zhi Neng medicine.

Zhi Neng medicine has a unique view of energy, stating that the cause of all ailments and illnesses is either a deficiency of energy or a condition of excess energy in the body. For recovery to occur, the energy in the fields must be adjusted. Such adjustments include self-adjustment and mutual energy radiation, when one is healing others. Energy can be developed in selected parts of the body by practising Dong Yi Gong. The speed and efficiency of healing is increased by developing higher energy.

Energy development in concert with the development of one's pureness or virtue (as expressed through Tao and Te) can open the door to communication with the universe or spiritual masters. Although this is not expressly stated in the book, it has been implied in many places that one can reach this state. Concerning the connection between Zhi Neng medicine and the theories of Yin/Yang and Five Elements, I believe that anyone having a basic knowledge of traditional Chinese medicine would be most interested in these sections of the book and benefit the most from them.

Fields and energy form the nuclei of Zhi Neng medicine. The most beautiful part and major focus of this book are the hand-fields healing methods and the Dong Yi Gong exercises. Therefore, a large portion of the book has been set aside to explain and provide instructions on these practices in very plain language.

To do hand-fields healing, you must be relaxed so that the body cells can vibrate and move freely as they are directed. Sound, mind energy and hand positions are used in the hand-fields healing methods to produce pressure gradients at different parts of the body. When doing this, the cell movements and the characteristic fields resulting from their movements can direct energy in the body towards achieving a balanced state and, ultimately, recovery from illness. This concept is completely in accordance with the scientific point of view.

Doing Dong Yi Gong is easy! Dong Yi Gong uses a lot of creative visualization, sounds and mantras, exercise theories and techniques. Anyone practising these exercises can develop energy, cultivate special skills, develop greater intelligence, strengthen the body and even communicate with the universe or spiritual masters. All one needs is patience, persistence and belief.

xi

In terms of my own experiences with Zhi Neng medicine, I have been most impressed with the hand-fields healing methods. Two years ago, I used to have chronic headaches that escaped medical diagnosis. I used the hand-fields healing method of *one hand near* my head and *one hand far* at my abdomen. In so doing, I visualized light flowing from the head to the Lower Dan Tian area. I silently read and repeated the sounds *yi-jiu, yi-jiu (1-9, 1-9)* for 3-5 minutes at a time. Gradually, the intensity and frequency of my headaches were much reduced. Eventually, my headaches disappeared. This has been most amazing to me.

I am most grateful to Master Sha for teaching his acupuncture technique to me. Compared to traditional techniques, Sha's Acupuncture Therapy is a much simplified method which uses significantly fewer acupuncture points. He concentrates energy and directs it through the needle, creating an explosive force that opens up the areas of accumulated energy to balance them. If necessary, Master Sha may consult the patient's soul to find out the actual problem, the best method of treatment, and the best time for treatment. Master Sha treats his patients with sincerity and compassion. Thousands of people have benefited from his revolutionary style of *energy-acupuncture* and experienced relief from their medical problems.

I am also impressed that before Master Sha teaches any of his disciples, he encourages them to purify their mind. Sincerity, passion, honesty, the cultivation of sympathy and a caring heart are qualities strictly demanded of them. As well, the practice of Dong Yi Gong is a must for development of the necessary energy which is the key component of Sha's Acupuncture Therapy.

I am very happy to have had the honour of reading Master Sha's book before publication and to share my impression in these few words. My hope is that anyone reading this book will receive the same benefits as I have from Zhi Neng medicine, and more. Read, follow, and have faith.

Wen-Hsiung Chen, Ph.D., Professor, Physics
Taiwan, 1996

Acknowledgements

First of all, I would like to thank my adoptive father and my master, Zhi Chen Guo, my adoptive mother, Jin Ying Jiang Guo, my adoptive grandmother and five sisters, for training me and supporting my work in Zhi Neng medicine. There are no words sufficient to express the depth of my gratitude and respect for them.

A very special thank you from the bottom of my heart goes to Sylvia Chen and her family for supporting Zhi Neng medicine for the past four years in Canada, the United States, Taiwan and China. Sylvia's energy, effort, contribution and commitment are deeply appreciated.

I thank Dr. Wen-Hsiung Chen, Professor of Physics at the National Chiao-Tung University of Hsin-Chu, Taiwan for his support over the years and for verifying the physics of Zhi Neng medicine.

I thank Dr. Faudry Pierre-Louis of Montfort Hospital in Ottawa for writing the foreword for this book. We first met when he attended my seminar on Zhi Neng medicine at Ottawa's International Academy of Natural Sciences in October 1995. Dr. Pierre-Louis has since become a great supporter of Zhi Neng medicine and is medical advisor to the International Institute of Zhi Neng Medicine.

I also thank Dr. Donald W. Stewart of Vancouver, BC, for fully supporting Zhi Neng medicine. Dr. Stewart is also medical advisor to the Institute.

Special thanks goes to Dr. W.P. Chang of the World Health Organization (Regional Office of the Western Pacific). I thank Dr. P.H. Gruner and Dr. Mark J. Yaffe of St. Mary's Hospital, Montreal, Quebec, for inviting me to St. Mary's to give a lecture on Zhi Neng medicine to more than two hundred doctors and nurses.

My deep appreciation goes to Cecil L. Rotenberg, Q.C., immigration specialist, and his wife, Miriam Leung Rotenberg of Toronto. Thanks also, to Dr. Stephen M. Reingold, medical oncologist at Peel Memorial Hospital of Brampton and Dennis Mills, MP (Broadview-Greenwood), of Ontario for helping me immigrate to Canada.

For their strong support of Zhi Neng medicine, I wish to thank Tony Yee, the publisher of *City Week* magazine, and Mr. and Mrs. George Lee of Vancouver, BC; Lorna J. Hancock, executive director of the Health Action Network Society of Burnaby, BC; Lady Dorothy Marshall, executive director of the International Academy of Natural Science in Ottawa; and Augusto and Honey Ednacot, Lilian Saw, Paul and May Wong, close friends in Toronto.

Many thanks to my students of Zhi Neng medicine for helping make this a better book. Special appreciation goes to Jim Chow and Diana Bennest who spent endless days and nights processing and editing my words. I deeply appreciate Diana's contribution and full-time commitment to Zhi Neng medicine. Thank you, Steven Wong, for keeping the energy flowing and for reading so well. For editing, I especially appreciate and thank Gail Franklin and May Chew. Thanks also to Charonne Soubolsky, Benedito José Da Silva, Bozena Sacha, Tammy Tran, Lou Bennett, Diane Lafrenière-Fox, Vimi Jain, Brigida Milne and Roseta T. Dance for supporting from their hearts. I also wish to thank Yuan Yuan for her dedication.

For designing and laying out the whole book, I thank Jim YC Chow for doing an excellent job. He has urged me many times to write it and supported my work in many other ways. He has given his life to me, to Zhi Neng medicine and the Way, forgetting sleep, food and friends in his relentless dedication. He has summoned all resources available to him in the production of this book. Every page has been touched by his soul and by his sweat.

I am truly grateful to May Chew for her unwavering support and full committment. Aside from working a regular job, she spent the last few weeks with almost no sleep in editing this book. Her effort and contribution move my heart. I deeply appreciate Gail Franklin for her contribution and for fully supporting Zhi Neng medicine. I also thank Diana Holland for her contribution in the final editing of the book.

In the Philippines, I appreciate my very close friends who have fully supported Zhi Neng medicine and my work. They are Mrs. King Ha Chua, Mr. and Mrs. Lucio Tan, Domingo and Shirley Chua, Jimmy and Sally Cheung, Lo Piak Ha, Mr. and Mrs. Steve Lim, Laura Lim, Mr. and Mrs. Tony Lim, Julita Co Tan, Go Sy Pian Pian, Benito and Ester Pascaul, Jorge and Elena Go, William and Billy Khu, Tony Ching and Go Sick Ha, and their respective families.

XV

With great reverence and respect, I thank Wu Yi Shi, my Buddhist master in Taiwan, and Da Jun Liu, my I Ching professor at Shandong University, China.

I give humble thanks to my wife, Qion Xi Luo Sha, my children, my parents and my in-laws for fully supporting my vision of Zhi Neng medicine.

Last, but not least, I sincerely appreciate the support of all my patients and friends who have supported Zhi Neng medicine. Thank you very much.

Thank you.

Zhi Gang Sha
Vancouver, BC
March 1996

Contents

Chapter 1
Basic Theories & Principles of
Zhi Neng Medicine

Chapter 2
Energy Development

Chapter 3
Energy Balancing and Healing

Conditions of the Mouth

Conditions of the Ear

Conditions of the Neck

Conditions of the Lungs

Conditions of the Heart

Conditions of the Spleen and Stomach

Conditions in the Liver and Gall Bladder

Conditions of the Kidney and Bladder

Conditions of the Lower Abdomen

Feminine Conditions

Conditions of the Blood Vessels

Cold Conditions

Conditions of the Bones and Joints

Skin Conditions

Conclusion

Appendix

List of Figures

List of Tables

Index

Introduction

Zhi Neng medicine, pronounced *"ju nung,"* is a revolutionary new health science from China that gives ordinary people the power to restore their own health and the health of others. Zhi Neng medicine literally translates as *intelligence* and *capabilities of the mind*.

The principles of Zhi Neng medicine were first introduced to the public in 1992 by Zhi Chen Guo, the founder of Zhi Neng medicine. Since then, Zhi Neng medicine has been widely accepted by the Chinese population because it is so easy to learn and effective in practice. Many supposedly incurable health problems have been solved by the use of Zhi Neng medicine, which has attracted the attention of western doctors, traditional Chinese doctors and other health-related professionals.

Zhi Neng medicine is a medical science and philosophy born of many different fields of knowledge. These include the ancient Chinese philosophies of Yin Yang, Five Elements, I Ching, Tao, Te, Qi Gong, Buddhism, Confucianism and traditional Chinese medicine as well as the scientific disciplines of western medicine, biology and physics.

Zhi Neng medicine enables you to be responsible for your own health. It will help you balance and develop your energy to prevent illness, relieve pain, stop illness in the early stages, and recover faster if you are already very sick. You can develop more energy. You can strengthen your immune system. You can prolong your life and improve its quality.

1

Zhi Neng medicine improves and increases your mind's capabilities. Developing the mind's latent power is important for improving ourselves as human beings. Besides relieving the symptoms of illness, Zhi Neng medicine develops enhanced memory, better comprehension, greater patience, deeper insight and heightened perception and intuition. The clarity of your thinking and your stamina will increase. Your awareness will be heightened, even to the point of developing precognitive and telepathic functions.

2

This book describes the basic philosophies, principles and techniques of Zhi Neng medicine to relieve pain and illness in yourself and others, and the skills to develop higher spiritual awareness. All you need is an open mind, patience and practice.

The Zhi Neng medicine flower has begun to open in the West. It will rapidly blossom throughout the world. It is my hope that you will learn and apply the simple techniques presented here and find Zhi Neng medicine to be effective in your life.

Welcome to Zhi Neng medicine!

Chapter One

Basic Theories
& Principles of
Zhi Neng Medicine

Background

Zhi Neng medicine was first introduced to the public on July 6, 1992, by Zhi Chen Guo, its founder. An audience of thousands in Tian Jing, China, listened as Master Guo presented his insights and techniques developed over forty years of study and practice in traditional Chinese medicine, Qi Gong, western medicine and his own extraordinary functioning of the senses. He had combined the principles of these four disciplines to create the new discipline of Zhi Neng medicine.

Zhi Neng medicine incorporates ideas from both traditional Chinese medicine (TCM) and western medicine to relieve ailments. Applied separately, both western medicine and traditional Chinese medicine have their respective advantages and disadvantages. When they are combined in Zhi Neng medicine, the world has a better and more encompassing medical philosophy for health and illness[1].

However, Zhi Neng medicine is more than just the combination of TCM and western medicine. The new discipline incorporates facets of ancient Chinese disciplines like Yin/Yang, Five Elements, I Ching, Tao, Te, Buddhism, Confucianism and Qi Gong. The Zhi Neng medicine concept of health considers spiritual health along with physical and mental health. The discipline of *soul study* is also an integral part.

The link between cellular vibration and health is what distinguishes Zhi Neng medicine from other medical models. This idea is central to Master Guo's perspective on Zhi Neng medicine *Cell Theory, Field Theory, Space Theory* and *Message Theory,* and the healing methods he has developed, including *One-Hand Healing, One Hand Near-One Hand Far,* and so forth.

---

[1] Tian Jing University, Tian Jing and Fu Dan University, Shanghai have researched Zhi Neng medicine theories and principles, proving that Zhi Neng Medicine is effective in restoring health and in strengthening the function of the immune and other systems in the body.

Guo's Cell Theory

Biology defines the cell as the smallest independently functioning unit of the human body. A cell consists of membrane, nuclei, cytoplasm, DNA, RNA, mitochondria and other organelles. Every internal organ and tissue in the body consists of cells. Living cells have various functions, such as protection, secretion, immune duties, reproduction, absorption, elimination, etc.

Western medicine studies biochemical changes in cells but does not pay much attention to cell vibration or cell energy with respect to health. In addition to performing its various functions, every cell vibrates. As well, cells are constantly expanding, contracting, spinning, wobbling, twisting and rocking. Some movements are consistent, others random. Any type of cell activity radiates energy. The concepts of cell vibration and energy are central to the principles of Zhi Neng medicine, and distinguish it from western medicine.

Consider brain cells as an example. The brain is the control centre of the central nervous system. Its messages tell the body how to operate and function, even down to the cellular level. A large number of brain cells vibrating in strong, healthy patterns will send strong, coherent messages to the body for better health and functioning. Brain research scientists estimate that the human brain has ~15 billion cells, of which only 10 percent are used. The other 90 percent are called *potential* or *dormant cells.*

Mind power is a function of the brain and the soul. Zhi Neng medicine considers that the mind is roughly 80% brain and 20% soul. Awakening more of the potential cells in the brain makes available more brain power. A stronger, more aware brain means a stronger, more powerful mind and greater abilities for everything. Similarly, mind power can also be increased by working on the spiritual richness of the soul.

How can the dormant cells in the brain be awakened? Physical exercise alone won't develop them. You need to use creative visualization, special sounds or mantras and hand postures. These techniques create the patterns of vibration necessary to stimulate the potential brain cells properly. With enough time and practice, the potential cells start to vibrate in response to these patterns. When this happens, your mind power increases and your body develops more energy.

Cells vibrate more strongly when you develop your energy. They also tend to vibrate in balanced patterns that support good health. When your cells vibrate strongly, they influence nearby cells to vibrate in the same way. This phenomenon, known as *sympathetic vibration,* encourages all the cells in your body to vibrate in the same healthy patterns. You can even encourage another person's cells to vibrate in accordance with your healthy patterns if your energy is highly developed.

Cell vibration is affected by many factors[2], some of which can cause either excess energy or insufficient energy to develop in the body. Both conditions adversely affect health. The body's energy patterns must be restored to relative balance to allow for recovery to occur.

Excess Energy

Too much energy in an area of the body is caused by over-active cells. Intense energy radiates from them and accumulates in the area. If the energy is too great, it cannot be transmitted fast enough to other parts of the body. This energy concentrates in specific areas and becomes *blocked.*

Imagine a river. The river level rises after a heavy rain. If there is too much water for it to carry away, the river starts to spill over its banks. Water then pools on the surrounding land and stagnates. Diseases start spreading. Energy can accumulate in the body in much the same way.

---

[2] Factors affecting cell vibration include the weather, emotions, stress, diet, environmental pollution, physical and/or mental trauma, injury, ill health, disease, infection, inflammation, and many other external and internal influences.

When energy doesn't flow properly in the body, conditions for infection and poor health are established. The result may be pain, inflammation, infection, hemorrhage, heart attack, stroke, cysts, unusual growths, tumours and hyperactivity of the organs. *Excess energy in any area of the body forms a high-intensity field.*

Insufficient Energy

Factors such as the weather, pollution and emotions can also cause cells to vibrate too slowly. The energy radiating from these cells will not be enough for healthy functioning. The symptoms of low energy may include *hypofunctioning* of the organs, fatigue, lowered immunity, degenerative changes, edema and weakness. *A deficiency of energy in any part of the body forms a low-intensity field.*

Cell Theory Application

The Zhi Neng medicine concept that health is related to cell energy radiation lets us see how both western medicine and traditional Chinese medicine are correct, even though they seem so different.

For example, let us consider a case of sore throat related to the common cold. Following are three perspectives on this ailment that show the differences and similarities amongst traditional Chinese, western and Zhi Neng medicine.

Traditional Chinese medicine (TCM) explains that a cold materializes when natural *Qi* (energy) from the environment invades the lung meridian, stagnates and turns into excess heat (yang). Treatment would involve a prescription of herbs to cool or balance the heat in the throat area. Acupuncture can be performed to remove the blocked *Qi* and to promote the proper flow of Qi in the meridians.

Western medicine says that the common cold is caused by a viral or bacterial infection. The body's cells and immune system have been invaded by pathogens. Where inflammation is evident, western doctors would give antibiotics to control the bacterial activity. In the case of a viral infection, patient comfort would be attended to while the cold took its course and the body developed antibodies. Additionally, medication could be prescribed to relieve such symptoms as headache, nasal congestion, soreness and coughing. *Western medicine does not normally consider the link between cellular vibration and health.*

Zhi Neng medicine's explanation of the cold includes concepts from both traditional Chinese medicine and western medicine. Zhi Neng medicine accepts western medicine's theory of a bacterial or viral infection. However, it goes further by considering that an infection would stimulate the throat cells to make them vibrate more than usual. Overactive cells radiate more energy than can be absorbed or dissipated by the neighbouring tissues and organs. The result is blocked energy in the throat, subsequently manifesting as a sore throat or inflammation.

9

Zhi Neng medicine also accepts the belief of traditional Chinese medicine that when too much natural *Qi* invades the lung meridian, it causes too much heat in the throat. Zhi Neng medicine considers that this heat will stimulate cells in the area to vibrate faster and radiate more energy than can be dissipated. Energy thus accumulates and becomes blocked in the throat. Once again, Zhi Neng medicine says that the sore throat is the result of energy blockage in the throat cells.

From the Zhi Neng medicine perspective of cell vibration, the interpretations of illness given by western and traditional Chinese medicines are both correct; they just explain different aspects.

Guo's Field Theory

Cells vibrate constantly. This constant cell activity radiates energy and creates a force field around the cells. Cells in the same tissue group radiate energy to form a characteristic field around that tissue. Each internal organ has its own field which is different in intensity from the fields of other organs.

The field theory of physics dictates that the energy in high-intensity fields will move to lower-intensity fields. Energy always flows from an area of higher density to an area of lower density until the energies in both fields equalize. Energy does not flow between fields which have the same intensity. Without energy flow, there can be no life.

Master Guo explains that *energy moves in the body in the same way — from higher-intensity fields to lower-intensity fields.* Energy flows through the body, either directly or through various energy channels known as *meridians*[3]. You are considered to be in good health if the fields in your body are relatively balanced and energy flows well. The more unbalanced the energy in the fields, the sicker or further removed from health you are.

High-intensity fields form in the body where excess energy has accumulated. This is due to the hyperactivity of stimulated cells, whose intense vibration generates more energy than can be dissipated. Examples of high-intensity fields in the body are areas where inflammation, pain, stiffness, growths, tumours or cysts occur.

---

[3] In traditional Chinese medicine, the pathways that energy flows through in the body are known as *meridians*. Traditionally, Qi is defined as the vital energy of the body. Anatomically, blood circulation pathways and meridians are not the same. Typically, *Qi leads and blood follows.*

Factors such as strong emotion can cause excess energy to build up in the body. For example, if you get very angry, your liver cells vibrate more strongly than usual. A high-intensity field forms around the liver, which affects other organs in the body. For instance, this excess energy may affect the stomach and cause a feeling of fullness, pain, poor appetite or indigestion. If the anger is not released, the liver cells will vibrate more and radiate even more energy. Over time, the excess energy accumulated may produce inflammation or a tumour in the liver itself or in other organs.

Low-intensity fields form in the body where cell activity is insufficient for proper functioning and health. This may be caused by many factors including emotions, weather, injury, pollution, chemicals, etc. The symptoms of insufficient energy are poor organ functioning, weakness, fatigue and poor immune system response.

Guo's Space Theory

There are many internal organs and tissues in the body. Each radiates energy and forms a specific field around itself. The fields of these organs and tissues interact with the fields of every other organ and multiple new fields are formed in the *space* where different fields meet. Some fields reinforce each other and increase in intensity, some cancel each other out or decrease in intensity, and others form different energy patterns altogether. The energy in the fields between the organs can strongly affect the organs themselves.

For example, the liver radiates energy and forms a field around itself; the stomach radiates energy and has its own field. The liver's field radiates to the stomach's field. The stomach's field radiates back and affects the liver's field. In the space between the field of the stomach and that of the liver, a new and third field forms. Any factor that makes the stomach cells vibrate too much will intensify the field between the stomach and the liver. This new field radiates back to strengthen and affect the fields of the stomach and liver.

Energy in the field increases. Poor health results if too much energy builds up in the *space* between other fields. Only when the excess energy dissipates can good health be restored. This may explain why some people still feel discomfort in the upper abdomen even when laboratory tests show no cause for their pain. The patient truly feels pain but there seems to be no clear reason. Zhi Neng medicine explains that *the patient may have a problem with excess energy in the field between the stomach and the liver.* A simple Zhi Neng medicine balancing technique can be used to solve this problem, by dissipating the highly concentrated energy and rebalancing energy in the fields of the body.

Guo's Message Theory

The sun radiates energy, in part as heat and light. The moon also radiates energy. Your cells radiate energy constantly. Trees, forests, oceans and rocks also constantly radiate energy. Everything in the universe radiates energy and sends out a message at the same time. Everything in the universe communicates with everything else. Most people are not aware of receiving these messages from the universe, but their subconscious mind knows.

If you develop your mind, body and soul highly enough, you can not only feel the energy, you can also receive the message. There is an area in the body that is known as the *message centre*[4]. The key to developing it is to fight your selfishness and develop your spirituality. You will be able to communicate with Jesus, Buddha, your spiritual guide, the universe, the sun, moon, planets, oceans, trees. Nothing will be hidden from you once you have reached this stage.

When you first open up your message centre, you will receive many incorrect messages. Accurate interpretation depends on many factors. These include the pureness of your character as well as the level of soul

---

[4] The message centre of the body is the Middle Dan Tian. It is one of the five key energy areas of the body discussed in Chapter 2.

development you have reached. Other factors include your readiness to receive messages, personality, natural energy and inherited factors. You must take the time and make the effort to develop accuracy in interpreting the messages. Do not force things or expect too much. Let it come naturally or you may harm yourself.

If your energy is developed highly enough, you will be able to communicate with your own organs and body tissues and send them healing messages. You will even be able to communicate with cells and tissues in other people to restore their health faster. You will also be able to understand the messages you are receiving. Suppose you have a weak heart and you smoke too much. Your heart may send out a message such as, *"Don't smoke because it hurts me. I feel uncomfortable. I can't breathe. Please stop or I'll stop."* A heart attack happens if you ignore the message long enough.

13

Yin/Yang Theory

The concept of Yin/Yang is one of the basic foundations of traditional Chinese medicine. This theory classifies all things into two opposite aspects — yin and yang. Yin/Yang is a universal law that governs all things, from the smallest to the largest, for both living and inanimate things.

Yin/Yang is a relative concept; it is not absolute. Everything can be divided into yin and yang. Any two things can be compared to determine which is yin and which is yang. Yin is the one with lower energy; yang, the one with higher energy.

Everything that has *fiery* characteristics belongs to yang. Fiery characteristics are hot and bright; they move upward and outward. They tend to be excited, fast and violent.

Everything that has a *water* characteristic belongs to yin. Water characteristics are cool and dark. They move inward and downward and tend to be slow and peaceful.

The Yin/Yang characteristic of *opposites* can be seen with some common Yin/Yang pairs, as listed in Table 1.

Table 1.   Common Yin/Yang Pairs

YIN	YANG
water	fire
woman	man
cold	hot
dark	light
passive	active
quiet	noisy
down	up
moon	sun
night	day
earth	heaven
winter	summer
soul	body

All the internal organs can also be put into yin or yang categories, as shown in Table 2. Yin organs are *zhang;* yang organs are *fu* in traditional Chinese medicine. Each internal organ has a corresponding organ which is its Yin/Yang opposite. Thus, the liver is yin, paired with the gall bladder, which is yang, etc.

Table 2.   Yin/Yang Organ Pairs of the Body

YIN (Zhang)	YANG (Fu)
liver	gall bladder
heart	small intestine
spleen	stomach
lung	large intestine
kidney	urinary bladder

The *interchangeability* of Yin/Yang can be seen in everything. Yin/Yang changes constantly. Yin and yang oppose each other, yet depend on one another for existence. They are always in relative balance; yin wanes as yang waxes, and vice-versa.

The Yin/Yang concept of *infinite divisibility* can be shown using the kidney. The kidney is yin relative to the urinary bladder which is yang. The kidney can be divided into kidney yin and kidney yang. Each kidney cell can also be divided into its yin and yang aspects. The membrane of the cell is yang, the nucleus is yin. Going further, the nucleus of each cell can be divided into its yin and yang aspects. Superficial parts of the nucleus are yang, the internal parts are yin. Anything can be divided endlessly into its yin and yang parts.

Time can be considered from a Yin/Yang point of view. For example, the Yin/Yang day is shown in Figure 1. Because night and day follow each other, they are inter-related and inter-changeable. Night and day are also inter-dependent since you cannot speak of one without the other. There is no night without day; there is no day without night.

15

The day is divided into 12 two-hour portions *(Di Zhi)*, each two hours covering the period when *Qi* flows most actively in the different organs and their meridians. These are the times when the organs respond best to medical treatment. (See Table 3.) For example, if you have a heart condition, the best time for treatment is during Wu time (11 am - 1 pm). Similarly, kidney problems respond much better to treatment during You time (5 pm - 7 pm). Zi time (11 pm - 1 am) is the time of the gall bladder meridian, which is related to the gall bladder; Chou time (1 am - 3 am) is the time of the liver meridian, which is related to the liver, etc. In China, this knowledge is called *Time Medicine.*

Table 3. Twelve Di Zhi (of the day)

Time	Name	Meridian
11 pm - 1 am	Zi	Gall Bladder
1 am - 3 am	Chou	Liver
3 am - 5 am	Yin	Lung
5 am - 7 am	Mao	Large Intestine
7 am - 9 am	Chen	Stomach
9 am - 11 am	Si	Spleen
11 am - 1 pm	Wu	Heart
1 pm - 3 pm	Wei	Small Intestine
3 pm - 5 pm	Shen	Urinary Bladder
5 pm - 7 pm	You	Kidney
7 pm - 9 pm	Xu	Pericardium
9 pm - 11 pm	Hai	San Jiao

In traditional Chinese medicine, yang represents fire and heat; yin represents water and coolness. You are healthy if Yin/Yang is balanced in the body. However, this is a relative concept. It is not absolute. If yin and yang were absolutely balanced, there would be no life. When they are unbalanced, illness occurs.

Too much yin in the body will appear as *cold syndrome*. You will feel cold, weak and tired. Organ functioning will be weak. Zhi Neng medicine considers this to be a condition of insufficient energy in the organ or body part.

Too much yang in the body will appear as *heat syndrome*. You will feel hot, flushed and feverish and your fluids may be deficient. Your organs or body will have too much *fire*, leading to inflammation or growths. Zhi Neng medicine would classify this as a case of excess energy in the body.

Yin/Yang imbalance in the body is corrected by taking herbs to cool the heat of excess yang or to warm the coolness of excess yin conditions. Acupuncture can be used to stimulate the flow of blocked or sluggish *Qi*. Following are some examples of Yin/Yang imbalance in the body and their interpretation through Zhi Neng medicine.

Inflammations, tumours and cysts are all considered to be a condition of too much yang and not enough yin. Zhi Neng medicine considers this to be a condition of accumulation causing energy blockage in the body.

Edema is a condition of too much yin and not enough yang. The Zhi Neng medicine view is that the kidney, lung and spleen organs may have low energy.

Kidney problems can occur with both yin and yang imbalance. Kidney yang is weak when the symptoms are cold feet and legs, no energy, impotence or premature ejaculation. Symptoms of weak kidney yin include dizziness and hot flushes without a fever. Zhi Neng medicine attributes both conditions to an imbalance of energy in the kidney.

Figure 1.

Twelve Di Zhi

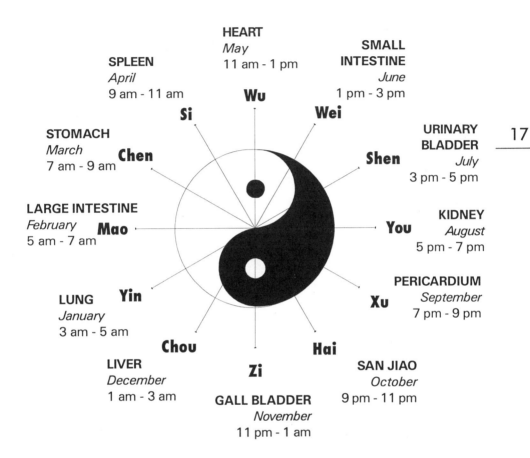

HEART
May
11 am - 1 pm

SMALL
INTESTINE
June
1 pm - 3 pm

SPLEEN
April
9 am - 11 am

Wu

Si

Wei

STOMACH
March
7 am - 9 am

Chen

URINARY
BLADDER
July
3 pm - 5 pm

Shen

LARGE INTESTINE
February
5 am - 7 am

Mao

You

KIDNEY
August
5 pm - 7 pm

LUNG
January
3 am - 5 am

Yin

PERICARDIUM
September
7 pm - 9 pm

Xu

Chou

Zi

Hai

LIVER
December
1 am - 3 am

GALL BLADDER
November
11 pm - 1 am

SAN JIAO
October
9 pm - 11 pm

KEY	**MERIDIAN** *Chinese Calendar Month* time most active

Notes:
- Each organ has a meridian (energy pathway) associated with it.
- Organs and meridians are most active in the time periods shown.
- Give healing and medication within the times shown for best treatment results for problems with the specific organs.
- The Chinese calendar is ~1 month behind the western Gregorian calendar.

Sore throat is a condition where too much yang or heat is in the throat. Natural *Qi* in the form of wind, cold and dampness moving by way of the meridians accumulates in the throat and changes from yin to yang. Too much yang accumulating in the throat area causes *heat syndrome.* You get well by taking yin character herbs to cool this heat. Acupuncture is used to promote *Qi* flow and to remove heat from the area. Applying Zhi Neng medicine techniques would help dissipate the excess energy radiating from the over-stimulated cells in the throat.

Five Elements Theory

The Five Elements Theory is another of the basic philosophies upon which traditional Chinese medicine and many other Chinese philosophies are founded. Together, Yin/Yang and Five Elements are considered the most important theories of the universe. The Five Elements Theory uses the idea of five natural elements to represent the characteristics of the internal organs and their relationships with one another.

The Five Elements are *Wood, Fire, Earth, Metal* and *Water*. In the human body, Wood represents the liver and gall bladder; Fire, the heart and small intestine; Earth, the spleen and stomach; Metal, the lungs and large intestine; and Water, the kidneys and urinary bladder.

Zhi Neng medicine looks at the theory of the Five Elements from the perspective of cell vibration and field intensities. The energies in the fields of the internal organs of the body radiate, support and control each other. They influence and affect each other all the time. If the energy in the fields of the organs is relatively balanced, you are in good health. If there is imbalance in any one of the organs, poor health results.

Relationships between the Five Elements are shown in Figure 2 and are generally of four kinds:

1. Generating (Mother/Son relationship)
2. Controlling
3. Over-Controlling
4. Reverse-Controlling

Figure 2.

Five Elements

Five Elements Classification of the Human Body

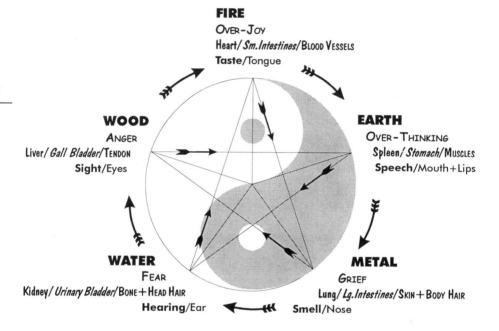

FIRE
Over-Joy
Heart/ *Sm. Intestines*/Blood Vessels
Taste/Tongue

WOOD
Anger
Liver/ *Gall Bladder*/Tendon
Sight/Eyes

EARTH
Over-Thinking
Spleen/ *Stomach*/Muscles
Speech/Mouth+Lips

WATER
Fear
Kidney/ *Urinary Bladder*/Bone+Head Hair
Hearing/Ear

METAL
Grief
Lung/ *Lg. Intestines*/Skin+Body Hair
Smell/Nose

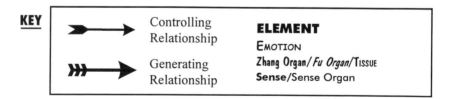

KEY

→ Controlling Relationship

⫸ Generating Relationship

ELEMENT
Emotion
Zhang Organ/ *Fu Organ*/Tissue
Sense/Sense Organ

Notes:

- In the *over-controlling* relationship, the organs follow the same order as that shown for the *controlling* relationship.

- In the *reverse-controlling* relationship, the order for the organs is the reverse of that shown for the *controlling* relationship.

- When the body is in good health and functioning normally, the *controlling* and *generating* relationships prevail amongst the organs. When the body is sick or in poor health, the *over-controlling* and *reverse-controlling* relationships prevail amongst the organs.

The generating and controlling relationships describe the normal physiological relationships between the internal organs when they are healthy and functioning properly. They generate and control each other to sustain harmonious and balanced conditions within the body. Zhi Neng medicine considers that energy is balanced and flows properly in the body when the generating and controlling relationships prevail.

The over-controlling and reverse-controlling relationships describe the pathological conditions between the internal organs when they are out of balance and functioning poorly or abnormally. When you experience illness, pain or poor health, it is because these relationships are occurring between the organs. Zhi Neng medicine considers that imbalances are caused by concentrated or blocked energy in the body.

The Five Elements Theory looks again at the example of sore throat related to a cold in the following descriptions of the relationships between the organs. Zhi Neng medicine considers that both conditions of excess yang (traditional Chinese medicine) and infection (western medicine) over-stimulate the throat and lung cells so that a throat infection develops. If very serious, this lung infection can radiate intense energy and even affect other organs. Clinically, complications such as bronchitis, pneumonia, and infections in the kidney, liver and heart have been observed in patients who first developed a sore throat after catching cold.

Generating Relationship

The generating relationship can be explained using the concept of a Mother/Son relationship. The Mother gives birth to the Son. The Mother produces, generates and nourishes the Son. Therefore, Wood produces Fire; Fire produces Earth; Earth produces Metal; Metal produces Water; and Water produces Wood.

Zhi Neng medicine considers that the internal organs radiate energy from cellular vibrations, forming their own distinct fields. The healthy functioning of the Mother organ *nourishes* the Son organ. Thus, the energy in the field of the liver irradiates and nourishes the heart; the energy of the heart irradiates and nourishes the spleen; the spleen nourishes the lungs; the lungs nourish the kidneys; the kidneys nourish the liver.

When the complications of a cold lead to kidney inflammation, traditional Chinese medicine says that this is a case of *the Mother transferring the problem to the Son* (Lung is the Mother of Kidney, the Son.) Some people with colds also experience poor appetite, nausea, vomiting, and diarrhea. This is an example of infection in the lungs affecting the stomach. *The Son gives the problem to the Mother*, and the order of the generating relationship is reversed.

Controlling Relationship

The controlling relationship shows the order of dominance or control governing the elements and the organs. Wood controls Earth, Earth controls Water, Water controls Fire, Fire controls Metal, and Metal controls Wood. This can be seen in nature where Wood draws nutrients from the Earth, Earth dams Water, Water puts out Fire, Fire melts Metal, and Metal chops Wood.

In Zhi Neng medicine, the energy radiating from an internal organ forms a field which radiates to and controls the field of another internal organ. The order of the Five Elements Theory says that energy in the liver field radiates to and controls the field of the spleen; the field of the spleen controls that of the kidney; the field of the kidney controls that of the heart; the field of the heart controls that of the lungs; the field of the lungs controls that of the liver.

Over-Controlling Relationship

An over-controlling relationship happens when one element subdues (over-controls) another and weakens it. For example, when Wood (liver) is very strong it *over-controls* Earth (spleen) and keeps it from functioning properly. If a cold leads to inflammation of the liver, TCM says that the lungs *over-control* the liver. *Metal over-controls Wood.*

In Zhi Neng medicine, when the field intensity of one internal organ is very strong, it will strongly radiate to the organ it normally controls. For example, Wood controls Earth, meaning liver controls spleen. If the liver is very sick and its cells are over-active, the energy it radiates creates a high-intensity field that affects the fields of the spleen and stomach. When this happens, people may experience a lack of appetite, poor digestion and abdominal gas.

Reverse-Controlling Relationship

A reverse-controlling relationship occurs when a controlled element is   **23**
too strong to be controlled by the organ normally controlling it. The natural order of the controlling relationship will be reversed, and the original *controlling* organ may be harmed.

For example, Metal (lung) normally controls Wood (liver). If Wood is too strong, Metal may not be able to control it. Then, the liver may rebel against the control of the lungs, and can even harm the lungs. Likewise, some patients with a cold can develop heart problems. If the excess energy in the lungs radiates to the heart, the heart muscle can become inflamed. This is an example of *Metal Reverse-Controlling Fire,* since Fire (heart) normally controls Metal (lungs).

Zhi Neng medicine knows that if the field intensity of one internal organ is too strong, it can radiate back and harm the internal organ which normally controls it.

For example, the liver field normally radiates to and controls the spleen and the stomach. If the spleen and stomach are very sick, their energies form very strong fields, which can radiate to, affect or harm the liver. This may result in a feeling of fullness in the abdomen and discomfort in the liver area. In this case, the controlling organ (liver) is not strong enough to control the organ (spleen, stomach) it normally controls.

Besides explaining organ behaviour, the Five Elements Theory can also be used to represent different aspects of the body, including the senses, tastes and emotions, and other things like colour, direction, the seasons, etc. Some of these characteristics are listed in Figure 2 and Table 4.

Senses

In traditional Chinese medicine, the senses are connected to various meridians. The Five Elements Theory says that the *liver opens on the eye, the heart opens on the tongue, the spleen opens on the mouth, the lung opens on the nose, and the kidney opens on the ear.* This means the liver meridian is connected to the eyes, the heart meridian is connected to the tongue, the spleen meridian is connected to the mouth, the lung meridian is connected to the nose, and the kidney meridian is connected to the ears.

The liver "opens" on the eye. Let us explain red and swollen eyes from the perspectives of traditional Chinese, western, and Zhi Neng medicine.

TCM regards the liver meridian as being connected to the eye and believes that red and swollen eyes are a symptom of too much heat (yang) in the liver. TCM would use herbs that have cold (yin) characteristics to cool the heat in the liver. Acupuncture can also be used to dissipate *liver fire*.

Western medicine does not recognize any relationship between the liver and the eye as they are anatomically separate and seemingly unrelated. Once obvious factors such as allergies, alcohol, lack of sleep, injury or colds are ruled out, swollen eyes due to bacterial infection would be treated with antibiotics.

Zhi Neng medicine agrees with TCM that red and swollen eyes are the result of too much energy in the liver area. Excess energy in the liver radiates to the eye and causes the eye problem. To determine the cause of eye problems, examine the liver and check for inflammation. Simple, effective Zhi Neng medicine theories, principles, techniques and methods can be used to relieve the eye inflammation (see Chapter 3).

Table 4.

Five Elements

Element	Yin Organ (Zhang)	Yang Organ (Fu)	Body Tissue	Finger	Sense	Emotion	Taste	Colour	Weather	Season	Direction
Wood	Liver	Gall Bladder	Tendon	Index	Sight Eyes	Anger	Sour	Green	Wind	Spring	East
Fire	Heart	Small Intestines	Blood Vessels	Middle	Taste Tongue	Excitable Over-Joy	Bitter	Red	Heat	Summer	South
Earth	Spleen	Stomach	Muscles	Thumb	Speech Mouth Lips	Worry Obsession	Sweet	Yellow	Damp	Late Summer	Middle
Metal	Lung	Large Intestines	Skin	Ring	Smell Nose	Grief Sorrow	Hot	White	Dry	Fall	West
Water	Kidney	Bladder	Bone	Baby	Hearing Ear	Fear	Salty	Blue⁵	Cold	Winter	North

Colour

The colour aspect of the Five Elements Theory is also listed in Table 4. The colour associated with the liver is green; the heart is red; the spleen is yellow; the lung is white; the kidney is blue[5]. This theory has been known in traditional Chinese medicine for 5,000 years, but almost no one uses the colour aspect of Five Elements Theory for healing.

Zhi Neng medicine uses Five Elements Colour Therapy to improve health. For example, if you have a heart problem, visualizing your heart vibrating or glowing with a bright red light will strengthen it. If you have a spleen or stomach problem, visualize the spleen or stomach area glowing and radiating bright yellow light. For lung problems, see both lungs radiating and glowing with brilliant white light. For kidney problems, visualize bright blue or purple light in the kidneys. For liver problems, think of bright green light pulsing and glowing in the liver.

You can also apply the colour associations of the Five Elements to your clothing, your food and your living space. For example, the strength of your liver will be reinforced by wearing green clothes and eating spinach and other greens. Wear yellow clothing, live in yellow rooms or eat yams to strengthen the spleen and stomach, etc.

Sound

The sound aspect of Five Elements Theory is also used for healing in Zhi Neng medicine. Different Mandarin Chinese words and sounds make the cells of different organs resonate and stimulate them. Stimulated cells generate and radiate more energy, becoming stronger in the process. When saying the sounds to strengthen a particular organ, visualize a bright light in its corresponding colour (Zhi Neng Medicine Colour Therapy) radiating, pulsing and glowing from that organ at the same time.

---

[5] TCM usually represents the kidney as being black in colour. However, the colour black is never used in Zhi Neng Medicine energy healing; doing so worsens your health condition.

The sound for liver is *jiao,* the heart is *zhi,* the spleen is **gong**, the lung is **shang**, the kidney is **yu**. If your liver is weak, repeat the sound *jiao* to increase liver energy; if your heart is weak, repeat **zhi** to increase heart energy; if the spleen and stomach are weak, repeat **gong** to increase their energy; if your lungs are weak, repeat **shang** to increase lung energy; if the kidneys are weak, use **yu** to build up energy there. The Mandarin Chinese healing sounds for the organs are listed in Table 5 below.

Table 5.   Healing Sounds for the Organs

Organ	Healing Sound
liver	*jiao*
heart	*zhi*
spleen	*gong*
lungs	*shang*
kidneys	*yu*

Summary

Five Elements Theory can be used to explain the relationship between the organs and how they affect each other. Understanding this theory can guide you to increase and balance your body's energy. Like the Yin/Yang Theory, the Five Elements Theory is a law of the universe which can be applied to many things.

Tao and Te

The spirit of *Tao Te* is exemplified by the quote *"In this life you plant a tree; in the next life you enjoy its shade."*

Tao is the way of heaven. *Tao* is the path of longevity and immortality. *Tao* is the source of heaven and earth. *Tao* is naturalness; *Tao* cannot be forced. Return to the pure state. *Tao* is a law of the universe.

Tao is the way.

To know the *Tao* in yourself, you must know and study Eastern philosophies and Western sciences. To understand the *Tao*, you must study not only the physical body, but also the mind and soul to uncover the secrets of the human body.

For example, *How long is a person's life?* Modern science cannot give you the answer. Life span is related to many factors, including your past lives and your present life. It is related to the environment in which you live, to your business and family relationships. It is related to how much you care about yourself. Living longer depends on you and your *Te*. If you have a high level of *Te*, your life can be prolonged.

Te, pronounced *"duh,"* is the record of your virtue. *Te* is the standard by which your soul is measured. *Te* defines the richness of your soul. *Te* is present in everything that you do. Every action in your past and present lives forms part of your personal record in the universe. At the end of this life, all your good and bad deeds are tallied, which determines how you return in the next life.

Your personal circumstances and health are also related to your *Te*. Think of the people you know who seem to be dogged with misfortune and others who cannot cure their illnesses or chronic pain. If *Te* is high, the conscious mind and physical body are in harmony and good health.

You can increase your level of *Te* by living every day with compassion and humility. Be kind and generous. Love unconditionally. Be sincere and honest. Help and care for others. Give of yourself. Work hard. Contribute. Fight your selfishness. Respect your family, friends, Masters, and every living thing. Change the way you live to increase your *Te* and spirituality.

29

Everything has a soul, living things and inanimate things too. If you highly develop your soul, you can communicate with family members, friends, saints and spirits, the sun, moon, earth, even a stone or a tree. Talk with a stone and it will answer you. Talk with the sun and it will talk to you. Ask God or Buddha for help and you will get a reply. Everything will talk with you if you can communicate.

A higher science of the universe is that of soul development. Like anything else, the soul needs food and seeks to communicate. In every life, the soul seeks knowledge; it may need healing. Know that *Te* is the single most important factor for developing your soul. Increasing your *Te* will help you to develop faster. Remember not to force it; follow the way of the *Tao* and let the soul develop naturally. Don't expect too much. Don't expect the Third Eye[6] or any special psychic powers to come to you. Doing otherwise can harm you mentally if your mind is not healthy and strong to begin with.

Developing energy with *Dong Yi Gong* opens the door to soul development. In the concept of *Tao Te*, *Qi* remains important for the body, but is not as important for spiritual development. Once the spiritual doors have been opened, *Te* becomes the most important key to the higher realms of the subconscious and the universe.

---

[6] Called the *Third Eye* by Buddhists, development of this energy centre in the body develops greater capabilities of the mind amd allows one to see beyond the plane of normal vision such things as auras and spiritual entities. Anatomically, the pineal gland coincides with the location of the *Third Eye*.

Feng Shui

Feng shui is mentioned here because the principles of *feng shui* affect your health, success and life.

The literal Chinese translation of *feng shui* is *wind* and *water*. These two elements are natural forces in nature. The concept of *feng shui* is energy and message. *Feng shui* is the ancient Chinese science that studies energy and message in relation to your environment. Health and success are closely related to *feng shui*.

Everything in the universe radiates energy and message. The energy and message surrounding your home affects your health. Many people get sick because the energy and message of their surroundings are not good for their health. Similarly, success in business and events in your life are also affected by the energy and message surrounding you.

Feng shui looks at the message and energy within the general vicinity of your home or office and how they affect you. This includes considering such factors as location, direction, architecture and floor plan, placement of mirrors, windows and doors, the surrounding trees, water bodies, mountains, spirits and field intensities, as well as other structures, facilities and operations relative to your space. All of these factors determine the resultant message and energy of your environment. Although you may not be receptive enough to understand the message and energy, they continue to act upon your body and subconscious mind. They are reflected in the health, happiness and success you experience in your life.

Zhi Neng medicine recognizes that healing is incomplete if the *feng shui* of the home and surroundings are not considered. Despite consulting the best medical practitioners for their illnesses, some people recover very slowly. This may be due in part to the patient's home *feng shui,* which affects the quality and speed of their healing.

Something as simple as changing the orientation of the bed may help in cases of insomnia. Chronic pain may be helped by removing items with harmful energies or making other adjustments in the home. A good *feng shui* master should be consulted to adjust the message and energy in your surroundings.

31

Feng shui principles are followed seriously in Asia and are only now becoming more popular and recognized in North America.

Chapter Two

Energy Development

Introduction

Energy is the force that radiates from the cellular vibration of living things, and the atomic and molecular activity of inanimate things. Traditional Chinese medicine defines *Qi* as *vital energy* or *life force*. Modern science and technology consider the work potential of energy. Western medicine uses energy in diagnostic equipment and for destruction of biological tissues. Zhi Neng medicine is founded on the principle that health is related to cell vibration and energy, and that energy must be balanced in the body for good health.

In human beings, energy radiates from cellular vibration. Developing higher levels of energy allows you to do more of everything. You will have more capacity for thinking, walking, talking, sleeping, growing, recovering from illness or pain, breathing, physical exertion, etc. To increase energy in the body and mind, you need to stimulate cell development. The energy levels of cells increase with higher development. Your body cells vibrate more strongly when you develop more energy. Zhi Neng medicine uses *Dong Yi Gong* exercises to develop more energy in the body and the mind.

Dong Yi Gong

Dong Yi Gong is the Zhi Neng medicine style of *Qi Gong, Qi Gong* being an ancient Chinese mental, physical and spiritual exercise for developing and balancing the energies of the mind, body and soul. The literal translation of *Dong Yi Gong* is *"using thinking exercise."*

This style of *Qi Gong* was developed by Master Zhi Chen Guo, the founder of Zhi Neng medicine.

35

Using creative visualization techniques, special hand postures and sounds, *Dong Yi Gong* allows you to quickly and safely develop energy in your body and mind. *Dong Yi Gong* can also be used to balance your body's energy when you are sick. Highly developing your mind with *Dong Yi Gong* will even enable you to distinguish energy imbalances in the fields of your body.

Dong Yi Gong exercises develop both the yin and the yang aspects of the mind and body. Some exercises are very fast, exciting and creatively stimulating (yang). Others are quieter, and more calming (yin). When you are practising *Dong Yi Gong*, cell vibration alternates between high excitation and slower stimulation. Energy will flow within your body with the creation of these areas of higher and lower energy density. The more and greater the Yin/Yang contrast you use in your meditation, the faster you develop. This explains why energy development is much slower with many other meditation styles that focus only on tranquillity.

The *Dong Yi Gong* exercises described in this book are very powerful experiences in creative visualization for developing your mind, body and soul. You will benefit most from them if you keep an open mind. Try to be creative and flexible. Make them work for you in ways you can relate to. You may want to read some of the descriptions aloud. If you are having trouble visualizing a golden ball, go and get one to look at. Substitute other images or ideas that work for you for the ones used in the visualizations. Repeat the exercises as often as you like. Remember to practice earnestly and patiently for faster energy development.

Five Important Energy Areas

In traditional Chinese medicine, energy flows through the body in 14 regular meridians. Six yang meridians feed into the *Du* meridian. Six yin meridians feed into the *Ren* meridian. The *Du* and *Ren* meridians feed into the *Zhong Mai* (Chong meridian), the most important meridian in the body.

Unlike traditional Chinese medicine, Zhi Neng medicine is not overly concerned with meridians for energy development. Instead, it focuses on developing energy in the five most important energy areas of the body as shown in Figure 3. The five energy areas which are key to developing greater capabilities of the mind and body are:

a)   the Lower Dan Tian,
b)   the Middle Dan Tian,
c)   the Upper Dan Tian,
d)   the Zu Qiao, and
e)   the Snow Mountain Area.

The locations of the five Zhi Neng medicine energy areas in the body are described using TCM *personal body inches*, referred to as *cun,* pronounced *"tsun."*

To find your *personal inch* measurement, bend your middle finger, and observe two creases on either side of the middle joint. One *cun* is the distance from the top end of one crease to the top end of the other crease (not the joint length of your middle finger.) One *cun* is also the width of the top joint of your thumb at its widest part.

Lower Dan Tian

Zhi Neng medicine regards the Lower Dan Tian[7] as the energy foundation area of the body. The Lower Dan Tian is a fist-sized energy centre that is found 1.5 *cun* below the navel, and 2.5 *cun* inside the body. This is the location of the middle of the energy centre. The Lower Dan Tian is considered the storehouse of the body's energy.

Middle Dan Tian

The Middle Dan Tian is also a fist-sized area, the middle of which is located 2.5 *cun* inside the body, starting from a point midway between the nipples. The Message Centre of the body, the Middle Dan Tian is the key to communicating with the universe. Developing the message centre is the key for developing your inner voice, your intuition and telepathic powers.

Upper Dan Tian

The Upper Dan Tian is a cherry-sized area located 3 *cun* below the Bai Hui acupuncture point. The Bai Hui is located at the intersection of a line drawn from the tip of your nose up to the back of the head and a line drawn from the top of one ear, up over the head, to the top of the other ear. In western medicine, the Upper Dan Tian is the area of the pineal gland. Taoists refer to this area as the *Ni Wan Gong*. Buddhists refer to it as the *Third Eye*. Developing the Upper Dan Tian is crucial to developing greater intelligence and capabilities of the mind.

Zu Qiao

The Zu Qiao, pronounced *"ju chow,"* is a cherry-sized area found just inside the bone cavity behind the *Yin Tang* acupuncture point (midpoint between the eyebrows). The Zu Qiao is similar in function to the Upper Dan Tian.

---

[7] The *Lower Dan Tian* is also the area where the soul usually resides within one's body.

Snow Mountain Area

The Snow Mountain Area is found by drawing an imaginary horizontal line straight through from the navel to the small of the back. From the back or the *Ming Men* (life gate) point, go in one-third of this distance and down 2.5 *cun* (just in front of the spinal column). The Snow Mountain Area is the most important energy area of the body, because the four most important meridians *(Du, Dai, Ren and Zhong meridians)* of the body meet in this area. The area gets its name from Buddhists who visualize a snow-covered mountain in the area.

39

Figure 3. Five Important Energy Areas in the Body

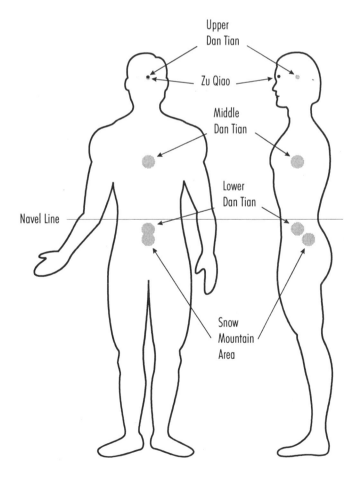

Energy Development Techniques

Zhi Neng medicine uses three key techniques simultaneously to develop energy in the mind, body and soul. *Hand positions* are used to create and induce fields of different intensities in the body. *Sound power* is used to stimulate the cells in the body to vibrate faster. *Creative visualization* trains the mind to concentrate and perform mental gymnastics in ways it may not be used to, and stimulates *potential* brain cells in the process. All three techniques are used at the same time in *Dong Yi Gong* to reinforce their effect on cell stimulation and energy development.

Hand Postures

There are many hand postures in meditation and Buddhist practice. Different finger positions develop energy in different parts of the body. The positions connect different meridians for proper energy flow and development. The finger positions are generally used in seated meditation. The fingertips do not usually touch. The following is a brief description of the more common hand postures and finger positions used in energy development.

a) *Finger Position I* The hands are relaxed and resting on the knees with the palms facing upwards. The fingers are slightly curved with the thumb and middle finger pointing to each other. This position develops the Upper Dan Tian.

b) *Finger Position II* Another variation of the first hand position is to point the thumb, index and middle fingers towards each other. The thumb should be pointing between the index and middle fingers.

The palms still face up and the hand is relaxed and natural, resting on the knees. This position is used to develop energy in the Snow Mountain Area.

c) *Opening Position* Both hands face palms up, with the right hand above the belly button and the left hand below the belly button. The distance between the hands is about one hand length and the hands do not touch the body. This position is used for starting standing-style Dong Yi Gong exercises and develops energy in the Lower, Middle, and Upper Dan Tian areas.

41

d) *Special Zhi Neng Medicine Hand Position* Close the right hand over the left thumb and make a fist. Close the fingers of the left hand over the right and rest the underside of both hands against the lower abdomen. Generally used for sitting-style meditations, this hand position develops energy very quickly in all energy areas.

e) *Prayer Position* The palms of both hands are brought up, facing each other but not touching, in front of the chest. The palms, fingers and wrists are relaxed and natural. This position is used for developing energy in the Middle Dan Tian, the message centre of the body. It is also used for stimulating and strengthening the organs.

f) *Lotus Face Position* Start with the hands in the *Prayer Position*. Bring them higher and open the palms to frame the face like a lotus flower. The base of the palms are a few inches below the chin. The hands are relaxed and do not touch the face. Use this position for developing intelligence and stimulating the mind. DO NOT use this position if you have high blood pressure.

g) *One Hand Near, One Hand Far Position* The *near hand* is 4"-8" (10-20 cm) from the body; the *far hand* is 12"-20" (30-50 cm) from the body. The palms of both hands face the body. Their relative distances from the body create fields of different intensities. This hand position is used for transferring energy in the body for balancing and healing purposes. *(See Chapter 3.)*

Sound Power

Sound carries energy. The faster you repeat the sound, the more powerful the energy. Sound energy stimulates cells in the body to vibrate faster. In Zhi Neng medicine, specific numbers and sounds stimulate various organs in the body. Some sounds are very powerful and can be used for developing energy in the body. These sounds can be repeated slowly, rapidly, quietly or loudly. Saying them rapidly stimulates the cells in your body to vibrate faster. Saying the numbers loudly stimulates the larger cells; saying them quietly, the smaller cells.

42

In Zhi Neng medicine, the healing numbers and sounds are said in Mandarin Chinese. Saying the numbers in another language will also result in healing because the message is in the numbers. However, the healing is more effective with the Chinese sounds because of their vibrational quality. For this reason, you will find, throughout the text, examples of how to pronounce them. In general, the healing numbers are listed first; the Mandarin representation and/ or phonetics follows in italics.

Mind Power

Along with the use of specific postures and sounds, Zhi Neng medicine includes *creative visualization* as part of its *Dong Yi Gong* practice to develop higher and more powerful energy in the mind. Training the brain with imaging and creative visualization techniques will awaken more *potential* brain cells, thereby increasing and improving mental capacity. Use creative visualization when you meditate to speed up the development of your mind and body as it is much more powerful than logical thinking.

You can also develop energy very fast by visualizing bright light in your energy centres. Try to visualize bright *white* or *golden* shining light. The brighter the light, the faster you will develop. If you have difficulty visualizing, persist. It takes time to develop this skill.

Standing Dong Yi Gong

For more details as required on all exercises, refer to the descriptions of the hand positions and Figure 3 for the locations of the energy areas in the body (pages 39-41).

The following are descriptions of standing-style *Dong Yi Gong* exercises for developing energy in specific Zhi Neng medicine energy areas of the body. Some are single exercises; others involve a whole sequence of positions. These exercises are performed standing up.

Developing Energy in the Five Energy Centres

Hand power, sound power, and creative visualization are used together in these single-sequence standing-style *Dong Yi Gong* exercises to develop power and energy in the five energy centres of the body. Repeat them as often as you like.

Key Steps

· Be relaxed.
· Aim the palms at an energy centre and imagine light glowing in the energy centre.
· Use the *One Hand Near, One Hand Far* hand position.
· Keep the fingers level; do not point them away from the body nor point them downwards.
· Repeat the sounds out loud (or silently) as fast as you can.
· Concentrate on visualizing the area glowing with light.
· Be creative and use your imagination to make the exercises work for you.

Lower Dan Tian

Energy development in the Lower Dan Tian will help you solve such problems as indigestion, constipation, and pain in the lower abdomen, as well as menstrual pain, weak kidneys, weak legs, etc.

- *Hands*: *One Hand Near, One Hand Far,* palms facing the Lower Dan Tian area.
- *Sound*: Repeat the sound *hong, hong, hong* or the number 9, *jiu,* pronounced *"Jew" or "Joe" (not Joey).*
- *Visualize* an electric bulb inside the Lower Dan Tian. Imagine it burning at 60 watts! 100 watts! 500 watts! 1000 watts! Visualize an explosion of light in your abdomen!

Middle Dan Tian

Highly developing this area will allow you to receive and communicate messages from the universe. The more you develop your Middle Dan Tian, the more sensitive you become to intuitive and telepathic messages.

- *Hands*: *One Hand Near, One Hand Far*, palms facing the Middle Dan Tian area. Alternatively, use the *Prayer Position (hand position e).*
- *Sound*: Repeat the sound *woo, woo* or *ah, ah.*
- *Visualize* a golden ball of light inside your Middle Dan Tian. The ball is constantly radiating brilliant, clear light.

Upper Dan Tian

Developing this centre increases your mind power. It benefits concentration, and helps people recover from senility and memory loss.

- *Hands*: *One Hand Near, One Hand Far*, palms facing the Upper Dan Tian area.
- *Sound*: repeat *wong, wong, wong* or the number 1, 1, *yi, yi.*
- *Imagine* a golden pearl in the Upper Dan Tian area. The pearl glows constantly with a bright, clear, golden light.

Zu Qiao

Developing the Zu Qiao helps develop greater intelligence and capabilities of the mind.
· *Hands*: *One Hand Near, One Hand Far*, palms facing the *Zu Qiao* area.
· *Sound*: *wong* or the number 1, 1, *yi, yi.*
· *Imagine* a very transparent, beautiful diamond in the Zu Qiao area, shining brilliantly, vibrating constantly, and causing the whole area to vibrate.

45

Snow Mountain Area

The energy radiating from the Snow Mountain Area supports and nourishes the brain. Energy from the Snow Mountain Area goes down in front of and enters the tailbone before moving up through the spinal column to the brain. Developing energy in the Snow Mountain Area will help you to overcome poor memory, quicken a slow response of the nervous system and relieve tinnitus (ringing in the ears), etc.
· *Hands*: *One Hand Near, One Hand Far*, palms facing the Snow Mountain Area.
· *Sound*: Repeat *hong* or the number 9, *jiu.*
· *Visualize* a snow-covered mountain in this area. Imagine a hot, powerful sun radiating heat and sunlight down on the Snow Mountain. The snow on the mountain starts to melt. Enjoy the beautiful, wonderful view. See and smell the melting snow turn to water. See energy rising as steam. The *steam-energy* rises up and nourishes your internal organs and tissues. Visualize energy going to all your internal organs or to any area needing healing.

Standing Dong Yi Gong Exercise Sequence

Perform this exercise as long as you like. Practising this sequence of exercises stimulates the mind and develops energy in various energy centres of the body.

Start with the *Basic Position* for standing *Dong Yi Gong* as described   **47**
below.

Basic Position

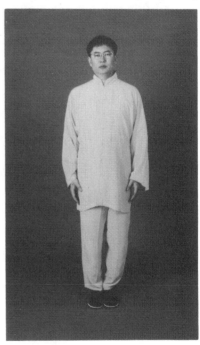

- · Stand comfortably
- · Contract your anus muscles slightly[8]
- · Touch the tip of your tongue to the roof of your upper palate[9]
- · Feet together
- · Knees slightly bent
- · Back straight
- · Hands at your sides
- · Close eyes slightly
- · Smile slightly
- · Relax

Basic Position for Standing Dong Yi Gong

---

[8] Relax the anus after the initial squeeze. The purpose of squeezing the anus at the beginning of *Dong Yi Gong* exercises is to connect the four meridians that cross paths in the Snow Mountain Area – the *Du, Ren, Zhong and Dai* meridians. Once the connection is made and the circuit complete, energy that develops during meditation can flow through all four meridians.

[9] Touching the tip of the tongue to the upper palate connects the *Du and Ren* meridians.

Position 1. *Opening to Receive*

- Step your left foot to the side (feet shoulder-width apart).
- Place your right palm 3" above the belly button (hand position c).
- Place your left palm 3" below the belly button
- Relax.

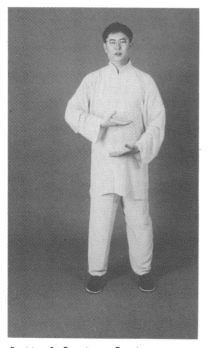

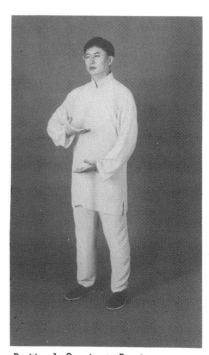

Position 1. Opening to Receive
(front view)

Position 1. Opening to Receive
(¾ view)

Position 2. *Energizing the Lower Dan Tian*

· Close your feet together (left foot moves back to the right foot).
· Place both palms over the belly button[10].
· *Visualize* a light bulb in the Lower Dan Tian area. See it burning at 40 watts, 60 watts, 100 watts; 500 watts, becoming brighter and brighter; 1,000 watts, 10,000 watts! Imagine an explosion of light! The whole abdomen shines and glows! It radiates brilliant, clear white light.
· Relax.
· Bring your hands down to your sides.

49

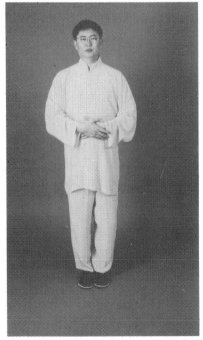

Position 2. Energizing the Lower Dan Tian

---

[10] Place both hands over the belly button. Men cover their left hand with the right. Women cover their right hand with the left.

Position 3. *Energizing the Zu Qiao* and the *Upper Dan Tian*

- Raise the arms straight out from the sides to shoulder level, palms forward.
- Turn your palms up, and bring your arms straight out in front of you.
- Bend your elbows and bring your palms to face you.
- Use *One Hand Near, One Hand Far*, palms facing the head area or the Upper Dan Tian.
- Visualize light glowing in the Zu Qiao and/or the Upper Dan Tian. Visualize bright light vibrating inside your head. Every brain cell is vibrating, fast and excited. See the whole brain as full of bright, clear light; radiating energy.
- At the same time, repeat *wong* or the number 1, *yi, yi.*

50

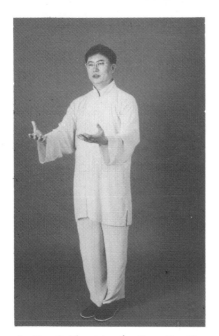

Position 3. Energizing the Upper Dan Tian and Zu Qiao

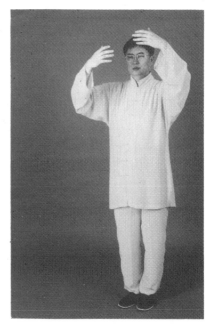

Position 3. Energizing the Upper Dan Tian and Zu Qiao

Position 4. *Energizing the Middle Dan Tian*

·   Move both palms down to face the Middle Dan Tian. Use the
    One Hand Near, One Hand Far hand position (see page 41).
·   Visualize brilliant light radiating in the Middle Dan Tian, the
    lungs and the heart.
·   Say or imagine sounds of energy like *whoo, whooo, whoo!!!*
·   See the Middle Dan Tian, both lungs and the heart vibrating
    with bright, clear light.
·   See your heart and your lungs as very clean, very healthy. When   **51**
    you have very strong energy in these parts it will help you to
    heal shortness of breath and heart problems of any kind.
·   At the same time, repeat *ah, ah, ah* or *woo, woo, woo.*
    These sounds will directly vibrate your lungs, your bronchial
    tubes, and your heart.

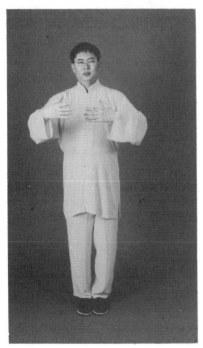

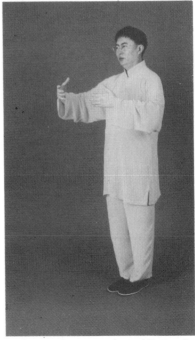

Position 4. Energizing the Middle Dan Tian
(front view)

Position 4. Energizing the Middle Dan Tian
(¾ view)

Position 5. *Re-energizing the Lower Dan Tian*

- Move your palms down to face the lower abdomen with the *One Hand Near/One Hand Far* (page 41, hand position g).
- Repeat *hong, hong* or the number 9, *jiu, jiu*.
- Visualize an ocean inside your lower abdomen. The ocean is churning, foaming, roaring! Let the fresh ocean waters cleanse your whole abdomen. Let it cleanse out your stomach, intestines, liver, spleen, urinary bladder, urethra, and any other part of your body that needs healing or cleansing.

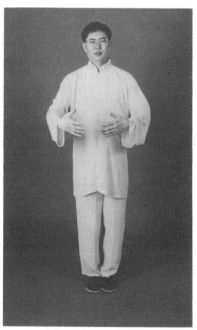 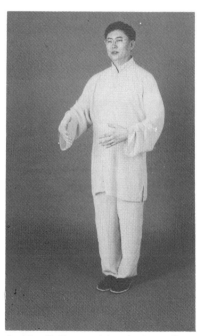

Position 5. Re-energizing the Lower Dan Tian (front view)

Position 5. Re-energizing the Lower Dan Tian (¾ view)

Position 6. *Invoking Higher Powers*

- Place your hands in the *Prayer Position*.
- Slightly close your eyes and focus on your fingertips.
- Repeat many times and rapidly *san san jiu liu ba yao wu* (3396815).

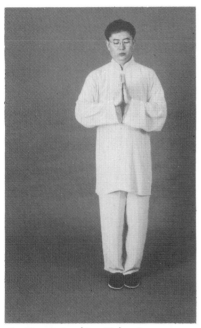

Position 6. Invoking Higher Powers
(front view)

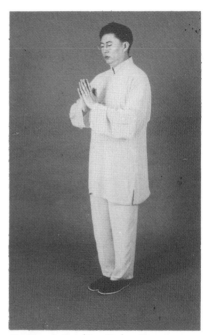

Position 6. Invoking Higher Powers
(¾ view)

53

Position 7. *Absorbing Energy From the Sun*

· Step your left foot to the side and stand with your feet shoulder-width apart, with *One Hand Near/One Hand Far*, holding your palms over the top of your head.

· Visualize sunlight shining down on you. It shines through you from your head through your whole body and out through your feet. The sunshine makes your whole body very warm, bright and transparent.

· Move your arms apart slightly, and tilt your hands to face the top of your head.

· Continue to imagine sunlight shining through your body. If any part of your body has a problem, imagine that part as very bright, shiny, clean and healthy.

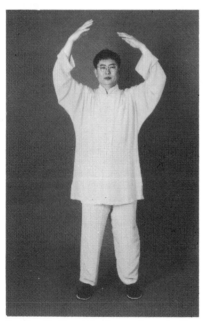

Position 7. Absorbing Energy from the Sun

Position 8. *Horse-Riding Stance*

·   Move your hands down to the *Prayer Position* (page 41, position e).
·   Squat down slowly, keeping your back straight and your thighs horizontal to the ground, heels and feet flat on the floor.
·   Run your tongue over your teeth and around your mouth to gather saliva.
·   Swallow and visualize the saliva going down to the Lower Dan Tian. Repeat three times.
·   Slowly rise to the *Basic Position* (see page 47).

55

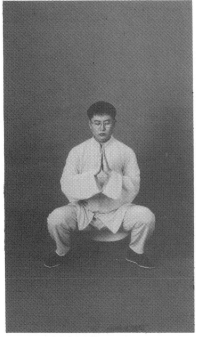

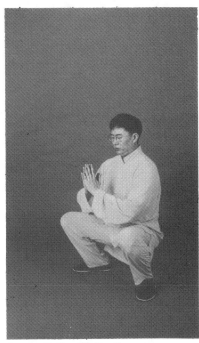

Position 8. Horse-Riding Stance
(front view)

Position 8. Horse-Riding Stance
(¾ view)

Position 9. *Returning to the Lower Dan Tian*

- *One Hand Near/One Hand Far* (page 41, position g); your palms face your lower abdomen.
- Visualize the whole abdomen glowing from the inside with bright, clear light.
- Silently repeat *hong, hong, hong.*

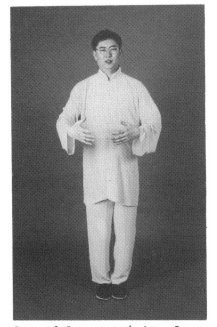

Position 9. Returning to the Lower Dan Tian (front view)

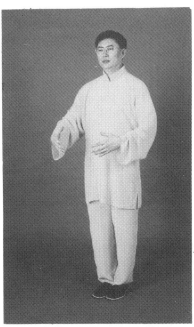

Position 9. Returning to the Lower Dan Tian (¾ view)

Position 10. *Visiting the Snow Mountain*

· *One Hand Near/One Hand Far* (hand position g), both hands
   behind you and palms facing the Snow Mountain Area.
· Visualize a snow-covered mountain in the Snow Mountain Area.
   Imagine a very hot, strong sun shining on the mountain. The
   snow is melting, and energy in the form of steam flows to any
   part of your body that you wish to nourish or heal.
· Lower your hands to your sides with the palms facing your body.

57

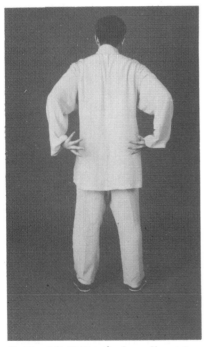 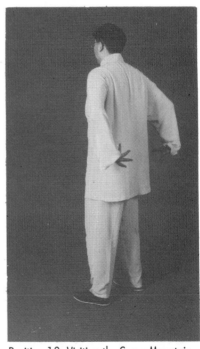

Position 10. Visiting the Snow Mountain   Position 10. Visiting the Snow Mountain
(back view)   (¾ view)

Position 11. *Energizing the Upper, Middle and Lower Dan Tian Areas*

- *One Hand Near/One Hand Far (hand position g)*, palms facing the Upper Dan Tian or head area. Inhale deeply and repeat *wong, wong, wong* continuously. When you say *wong* visualize the whole brain glowing with clear, *red* light.
- *One Hand Near/One Hand Far*, palms facing the Middle Dan Tian or chest area. Repeat *ah, ah, ah, ah* and visualize your whole chest glowing with clear, *white* light.
- *One Hand Near/One Hand Far*, palms facing the Lower Dan Tian or lower abdomen. Repeat *hong, hong, hong* and visualize your abdomen glowing with clear, *blue* light.
- Repeat many times.

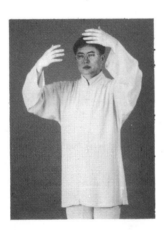

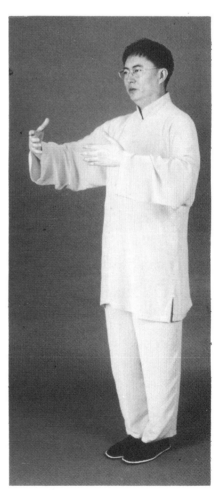

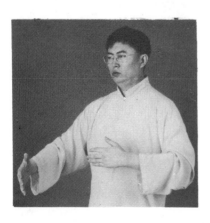

Position 12. *Healing With A Golden Ball In the Abdomen*

- Place both palms[11] on your navel.
- Bring your feet together.
- Imagine bright, cosmic light shining down on you from above.
  Feel the energy flowing through your head to your Lower Dan Tian.
- From below imagine bright light (the energy of the earth) flowing
  up through your feet to your Lower Dan Tian.
- Visualize a golden ball spinning inside your lower abdomen.
  Concentrate on the ball, and enjoy its beautiful, powerful, clear
  gold light. Spin it. Spin it faster. Your whole body feels very strong.
- Lower your hands to your side, with palms the facing the body.
- Relax.

59

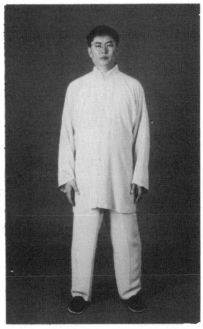

Position 12. Healing with a Golden Ball in
the Abdomen

---

[11] Men cover their left hand with the right. Women cover their right hand with the left.

Sitting Dong Yi Gong

Sit comfortably when doing these sitting-style *Dong Yi Gong* exercises as you may be meditating for hours. Repeat the exercises and perform them as often as you like.

When sitting on the ground, you can be kneeling, sitting cross-legged or in the half-lotus or full-lotus positions. When you are sitting in a chair, your feet should be flat on the ground, ankles and legs not crossed; your back should not be touching the back rest. Relax the whole body. Assume a hand posture. Touch the tip of your tongue to the upper palate[12]. Begin meditating and enjoy.

You may want to start by reading the visualization descriptions out loud. The discussions will give you a better idea of what the exercises are meant to do. Be creative and open-minded. Let your body flow with the experiences. Do not be alarmed if you feel your body responding strangely as you do these exercises. Body responses such as laughing, crying, shaking, or experiencing a hot, cold or tingly feeling simply mean that your body energy is changing and developing.

---

[12] Touching the tip of the tongue to the upper palate connects the *Du and Ren* meridians and lets energy flow through them.

Seated Positions and Hand Postures for Sitting-Style Dong Yi Gong
(Refer to pages 40 and 41 for descriptions of other finger and hand positions)

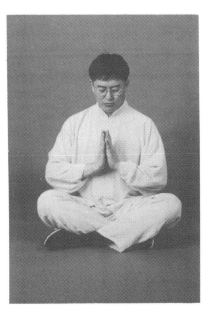

Cross-legged. Prayer Position (e)

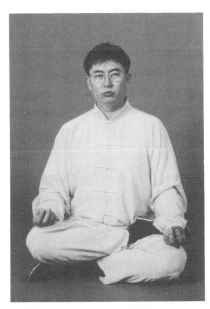

Half-lotus. Finger Position II (b)

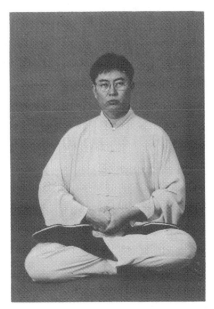

Full-lotus. Special Zhi Neng Medicine
Hand Position (d)

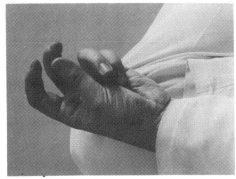

Detail - Finger Position II (b)

The Raging Sea

Visualize an ocean inside your lower abdomen.

The water is clear.

The sun is warm.

The view is gorgeous!

Breathe deeply. Feel the energy.

The tide laps gently, from left to right.

The breeze flows, swirling left to right, left, right

Waves are lapping. The wind picks up. Dark clouds.

Waves chop.*SLAPPING!* Whitecaps foam. Wind Howwwllls!

Wha! Wha! WooOO! Whoosh! WHOOSHHH!!

RAIN!!! THUNDER! LIGHTNING!!   WIND !!!

WHIP! WHIP! SNAP!! CRACK! ZAP!!! ZAP!!!

TSUNAMI!!   HURRICANE!!!   TYPHOON!!

The whole ocean is Churning! Boiling! *Raging !!*

Waves are smashing! Thunder roars!

S l o w l y t h e w i n d d i e s

t h e r a i n t a p e r s

s k y c l e ars

quiet

calm
time
time is endless

Discussion

Yin decreases and yang increases as the calm sea turns into a raging typhoon. Yang decreases and yin increases as the storm passes over the ocean and dies down.

Visualizing the boiling sea in your abdomen stimulates various organs, making their cells more active. Cell vibration increases and radiates intense energy. The field generated will strengthen the organs in your lower abdomen and nourish the organs of your other meridians.

This exercise is an example of how strong Yin/Yang contrast is used to develop energy in the body and mind very quickly.

Repeat this exercise many times.

Five Coloured Horses Galloping Up the Mountain

Visualize yourself and a horse on a plain, at the base of a mountain located inside your lower abdomen.

RED HORSE
On an open plain
Jump On in your RED robes
Walk the horse *dinga dinga dinga*
Trot Trot *dinga dinga dinga dinga dinga*
Canter *dinga up dinga up dinga up dinga*
GALLOP towards the mountain *dinga dinga*
GALLOP *up* the mountain counterclockwise *dinga*
higher higher faster faster faster up up up up
RED horse is SWEATING! STEAMING! PANTING!
SNORT! Whh-ee-ee! MUSCLES RIPPLE !! POWER!
GALLOP OUT ONTO THE TOP OF YOUR HEAD !!!
•
Stop
Rest a bit
Enjoy the view
Sitting on your horse
Turn the horse around
Jump back inside your head
RED horse starts walking clockwise
Trot Trot *dinga dinga dinga dinga dinga*
Canter Canter *spiralling clockwise down dinga*
GALLOP down the mountain *dinga dinga*
faster faster faster down down down *dinga dinga*
What is that you see in the distance? RED... A RED HEART!
GALLOP the HORSE STRAIGHT INTO YOUR HEART!

Discussion

This fast action-packed exercise develops energy in the five most important internal organs of the body.

As you ride your horse and spiral up the mountain, the energy developed in your lower abdomen radiates upwards to stimulate your brain. The increased cell activity increases energy in the brain. Coming down the mountain, the brain energy stimulates the internal organs to increase their energy.

Repeat the exercise for the *yellow, white, blue* and *green* horses. Wear robes of the same colour as the horses. You and the *yellow* horse will gallop in a counter-clockwise spiral up the mountain, pop out of your head, stop for a moment to catch your breath, race back down the mountain in a clockwise spiral and gallop at full speed straight into the spleen. Similarly, ride the *white* horse into the lungs, the *blue* horse into the kidneys, and the *green* horse into the liver.

The red horse strengthens the heart, the yellow horse strengthens the spleen, the white horse strengthens the lungs, the blue horse strengthens the kidneys, and the green horse strengthens the liver.

Ginseng Tree Growing On the Chong Meridian

Visualize a ginseng seedling growing into a tree inside your lower abdomen.

Ginseng seedling
  In the Snow Mountain Area
Tender shoots reach up
    A trunk grows in your spine
      Young roots spread down to your feet
        Your arms are branches, your legs are main roots
          Standing sturdy, strong, rooted on fertile Earth
Ginseng tree branches grow and fill your head
  Reaching to the Sun - *warm, golden, healing light*
    Bask in the *radiance* as the Sun nourishes your leaves
      Leaves rustle music above your head, *winking* gold in the Sun
        Your many fruits feel *light* and rich in the breeze
Take energy from the Earth !
  Take energy from the Sun !
    Make life force energy !
Send glowing *energy* to all parts of your ginseng tree
  Feel the strength, the vitality, the life in your veins
    Feel *energy glowing, flowing* all through your body
      Nourish all parts from smallest root to topmost branch
All your organs are healthy, strong, and vibrant !
  Your roots are bright, shiny and clean
    Your trunk is a glowing golden stalk
      Your branches are golden vibrant limbs
        Your leaves shine gold and blinding in the Sun
          Your fruits are heavenly golden orbs of *energy*
Everything radiates light and energy
  You shake with this energy! Vibration!
    Feel *STRONG* as the Sun smiles on you
      Bend and sway with the Wind
        Rejoice in your strength
          Relax

Discussion

The Chinese aptly call ginseng the *man root*. Ginseng roots truly look like miniature humans. *Ginseng nourishes Qi and blood.* This is why ginseng is the most revered herb in the East.

67

This visualization is particularly powerful as *you* are the one growing the ginseng tree inside yourself on the *Zhong Mai* (Chong Meridian). Your mind determines how big, strong, and powerful the tree is.

As the tree, you are rooted in Earth; energy from the Earth and the Sun flow through you, nourishing you. Feel the strength and vitality of the ginseng tree; draw upon its powerful healing properties as its *energy* runs through your veins and organs. Send this energy through the Zhong Mai to nourish and strengthen the rest of your body and organs.

Finding the Pearl at the Bottom of the Sea

Visualize an ocean inside your lower abdomen.

There is an ocean inside my tummy
Cool waters are clear blue silk
Smooth as glass

Look deep

Down

D
o
w
n
.
.
.
.
.
!
Oh!
Look!
A pearl!
A *golden* pearl!
At the bottom of the sea!
Glowing!   Pulsing!
Bright!   Golden!
Beautiful   Perfect
Shining   Pure
Strong!   Brave!
Beacon   Light
How lovely   Just to see
This little jewel!

Discussion

Concentrate on seeing the pearl at the bottom of the ocean for at least half an hour. It is radiating pure, golden light, and its beauty and energy takes your breath away.

This exercise directly develops energy in the *Lower Dan Tian* and *Snow Mountain Areas*, and indirectly develops the *Zu Qiao,* and *Upper Dan Tian* (Third Eye) energy areas.

Focusing on the pearl stimulates the cells in the *Snow Mountain Area*, which rapidly develop intense energy. This energy radiates to the brain and helps to develop more of the potential brain cells. Working with the *Snow Mountain Area* is a safe, easy and effective alternative to exercises that work directly on the Third Eye.

Seeing Yourself In Your Lower Abdomen

Visualize burning fires boiling a lake located at the bottom of your abdomen.

FLAMES burn brightly at the bottom of Snow Mountain
      Leaping higher and higher
      Boiling Lake above
YOUR SMALL PERSON
      Sits placidly
      Calmly
      On a lotus flower
      On top of a Red Heart
FLOATING in the middle of Boiling Lake
      Gases explode from the depths
      Whorls of mists tumble and roll
      Water hisses all around
YOU are serene
      Tranquil
      GLOWING!!
      Your body, your organs
      All shine brilliantly
      WHOLE
      STRONG
      HEALTHY
      Clear! Translucent! Pulsing!
YOU are serene
      Sitting on your lotus flower
      In this maelstrom of incredible energy
      Where the Universe ROARS! RUMBLES!
      The water ROILS! BOILS! SPITS!
      The flames CRACKLE!
YOU are serene

70

Discussion

The I Ching and Five Elements Theories are strong in this visualization.

Water is Yin; Fire is Yang. Water represents the Kidney; Fire represents the Heart. Kidney Water goes *up* to nourish the Heart and gives it Yin. Heart Fire goes *down* to nourish the Kidney and gives it Yang.

The elements, Water and Fire, nourish, coordinate and balance each other. When Fire is burning and Water is boiling, Yang and Yin are both excited. Yin/Yang is most changeable at this moment.

Your SMALL PERSON sitting serene in the middle of all this energy is your subconscious mind. See the SMALL PERSON as your soul. The lotus flower image has special significance and power. Visualizing your SMALL PERSON and your SMALL PERSON's organs glowing with *health, wholeness and strength* sends the same message to your subconscious mind, which will translate it into reality in your physical body.

Flashing Images Inside Your Lower Abdomen

Visualize anything you want inside your lower abdomen.

Watch ocean waves ripple in
The sun rising over the mountains blinds you
Pine trees sway overhead
Flowers waving madly
    The smiling face of a loved one
    Laughing children
    Swirling autumn leaves
    Rolling clouds of fog
Rushing mountain waters
Golden temples and cymbals
Leaping schools of dolphins
The sky dark with a thousand birds
Mist swirling off the ground in the early morning
    A kiss
    A puppy's joy
    The sheen of oil on a puddle
    A glance from across the room
    Your home
Rain dimpling a lake
The colour of pleasure
Coming home with your newborn child
Wheat fields under blue skies
    Dewdrops like crystals in the Sun
    Volcanoes gushing fiery lava
    A gleaming metal structure
    Ancient civilizations
Heaven ...

72

Discussion

Visualize anything and everything that comes to mind. See the images sharply and clearly inside your lower abdomen.

73

Open yourself to the feelings they bring. Switch images and scenes as *quickly* as you can.

Changing images quickly stimulates vibration of the brain cells and develops·mind power very quickly.

Three Dragons Playing with a Golden Pearl

Setting

There is a brilliant golden *Pearl* in your Lower Dan Tian
Green Dragon on the left. *Blue* Dragon on the right.
Yellow Dragon has its tail in Snow Mountain Area, body in front of your spine,
    head in your brain.

Catch Pearl (the game)

74

Pearl jumps up and down
Green Dragon jumps! Blue Dragon jumps! *jump jump jump*
Green Dragon sucks in Pearl.
Spits out Pearl...*gold dust everywhere*
Blue Dragon *flies* after Pearl. Catches Pearl. Spits out Pearl.
    Whoosh!! Green Dragon chases. Catch Pearl! Spit out Pearl!
    Zooo o o m! Catch! Spit!!! Swoop! Faster! Suck! Spit! Suck! Spit! Spin!
    What fun! Wee- ee-e! Hee-hee! Wonderful game!!

The Yellow Dragon's Ecstasy

    Oops!
Pearl jumps into Yellow Dragon's tail
bump bump bump de bump up Yellow Dragon's tail
    Oh joy! To have a golden peeaarrrrl in my tail!
    Wonderful! Now up my back! Squirm Squirmm m m with ecstasy . . .
Pearl Glows Blinding Hot! Pulse! Pulse! Pulse! Glow!!!
    I feel very warm! Purrrrr!
    Ahh hh h! shiverrr r y delight !!!
    Pearl is in my neck! in my mouth!
    Twitch! Spasm! Shiver my bones! Ooh h h! How lovely!
Pt-too-ee!
SPIT OUT PEARL! SUCK IT IN !!! *SPIT! SUCK!*
SPIN! *Pearl spins Whhrrr rr r r r whirrrrrr weee wee*
Pop!
Back into Yellow Dragon's mouth and down his body!
    Wiggle! Jiggle! Sigh! Lovely! Ahhhh!
Pop!
Pearl hops out of Yellow Dragon's tail

Catch Pearl again

Green Dragon snatches Pearl in his mouth
    Mine! Let's play "Catch" again.

Discussion

The Green Dragon represents the liver; the Blue Dragon represents the kidneys. Green and Blue Dragons flying around inside the lower abdomen increases the energy of the liver, kidney and lower abdomen.

This increased energy moves and flows through the Zhong Mai (Chong meridian) when the Pearl inches its way up the Yellow Dragon's body. More energy in the Chong meridian feeds and strengthens all the other internal organs because it is connected to all the other meridians in the body.

Chapter Three

Energy Balancing and Healing

Introduction

Zhi Neng medicine considers unbalanced energy in the body as the cause of illness. The disturbance can be either too much energy or not enough energy in one part of the body relative to the other parts.

Master Guo's Cell Theory discussed how every internal organ radiates energy due to cellular vibration. The energies in the fields of different internal organs interact with each other. The energy is always in a state of flux. When the organs are healthy, the energy in the fields between them is in a condition of relative balance; when the organs are ill, the energy in the fields is unbalanced. As a result, the intensities of the fields are also unbalanced.

Too much energy occurs when something stimulates the cells of an internal organ or a specific part of the body to vibrate too much and radiate much more energy than usual. As a result, energy around the area becomes highly concentrated and an energy imbalance forms between this area and the other parts of the body. Conversely, other factors can cause insufficient energy, which decreases cellular vibration and creates a much lower intensity field in that part of the body relative to other parts of the body.

Your body's energy and field intensities must be relatively balanced for recovery to occur. You can balance them by using simple self-healing techniques of Zhi Neng medicine to direct and transfer energy from areas of high intensity to areas of lower intensity. When energy flows, the energy blockage is removed. Pain is relieved, weak parts are strengthened, and health will be restored. You can balance energy in yourself and in others.

Zhi Neng medicine's healing techniques have helped to relieve chronic pain, joint pains, inflammation, headaches, fibromyalgia, fatigue, arthritis, asthma, and many other ailments. Critical situations can be improved with the use of Zhi Neng medicine. For example, patients have seen remarkable progress and recovery from stroke-related paralysis. Cancer, tumours and growths have been reduced. Patients with Acquired Immune Deficiency Syndrome have reported increased energy and respite. In general, people who practice Zhi Neng medicine are pleased with the improvement in their health.

Self-healing is simple to learn and will be more effective the higher you develop your body's mental and physical energy. Initially, results may be slow if you have a low energy level, but they will increase in speed as you develop more energy.

As with any other healing method you try, give Zhi Neng medicine a fair trial. Do not expect chronic pain that took several years to develop to disappear after a few healing sessions. Just as you don't expect antibiotics or medication to work instantly, use Zhi Neng medicine with the same attitude.

Be patient. Practice self-healing and energy development regularly, and you will see and feel a difference in your health.

Energy Balancing Techniques

Zhi Neng medicine's energy balancing techniques are the same as those used for energy development (Chapter 2). Energy balancing also makes simultaneous use of the three key techniques of hand positions, sound power and mind power or creative visualization. You can practice these techniques on yourself. You can also apply them to your family and friends to help relieve pain or illness.

Hand Postures

Hand postures are used to create and induce fields of different intensities around the body. Energy will naturally flow from an area of higher energy density to one of lower energy density. This is how a condition of relative energy balance is created in the body.

Zhi Neng medicine uses hand positions to increase or balance fields in specific ways. There are three main hand positions for energy balancing and healing:

a)   the palms face the body
b)   the fingers point to the body
c)   one finger points to the body

Palms facing the body are used in the *One Hand Near, One Hand Far Healing Technique*. The palms help direct and transfer energy from one part of the body to another. The palm distances of the *near hand* and the *far hand* relative to the body create fields of different intensities. Energy in the higher-intensity field created by the *near hand* flows to the lower-intensity field created by the *far hand*.

Never send energy away from the body by directing the palm outwards or away from the body as this will weaken you[13].

Pointing fingers to the body creates a higher, more intense field between the fingertips and the part of the body the fingers point to. This field has more intensity than a field formed with a palm (which is more diffuse). It is used in situations where energy is to be dissipated from a given area.

Pointed fingers are often used in the *One Hand Healing Technique* and sometimes in the *near hand* of the *One Hand Near, One Hand Far Healing Technique.*

Of all the hand positions used for healing, the highest intensity field is created with one finger pointing at the body. A very narrow, highly concentrated field forms between the pointed finger and the part of the body it points to. When the middle or index finger of the *near hand* is pointed in the *One Hand Near, One Hand Far Healing Technique*, it directs energy to move away from the body part that the finger is pointing to. The pointed finger is used to dissipate energy from highly accumulated areas such as tumours, cysts, swollen lumps and inflammations in the body.

Sound Power

Zhi Neng medicine uses the Mandarin[14] pronunciation of numbers and sounds to develop energy and to balance energy for health. Repeating different numbers aloud makes them vibrate and resonate different parts of the body. These sounds stimulate cell vibration; the flow of energy in the area increases, and enhanced energy and better health results. The numbers and the parts of the body they stimulate are shown in Table 6.

[13] Exceptions to never sending energy away from the body exist and usually involve critical situations where excess energy in a body part must be quickly reduced *(eg. inflammation of the aorta)*.

[14] The Mandarin Chinese pronunciation of the numbers and healing sounds used in Zhi Neng medicine work best for healing and energy development as described. Because the message is associated with the meanings as well as the sounds, saying them in another language still sends healing messages to stimulate the organs, but with less effect than if they were said in Mandarin.

Table 6.   Healing Numbers of Zhi Neng Medicine

Number	Mandarin	Pronunciation	Area Stimulated
1	*yi*	*ee*	head, brain
2	*ar*	*arh*	heart
3	*san*	*san*	chest, lungs
4	*si*	*sŭ*	esophagus
5	*wu*	*woo*	stomach, spleen
6	*liu*	*lū* (like *ewe*)	ribs
7	*chi*	*chee*	liver
8	*ba*	*bah*	navel, bellybutton
9	*jiu*	*jō* (like *joe*)	lower abdomen
10	*shi*	*shir*	anus
11	*shiyi*	*shir -ee*	limbs, hands, feet, legs, etc.

The *single sound* is repeated out loud for *developing energy* in the various organs and parts of the body.

For example, if your heart feels weak, you would continuously say *AR, AR, AR, AR, AR* (2,2,2,2,2) while visualizing your heart pulsing with bright red light. Saying the sounds sharply and quickly would stimulate your heart cells to vibrate faster and radiate more energy (e.g. ar, ar, *AR, AR, AR, AR).* Saying the sounds in a long, sonorous tone produces a gentler effect (e.g. *A A A A A A R R R RR,A A A A A A R R R RR ...*)

A combination of *two or more* number sounds in Zhi Neng medicine healing is used for *transferring energy* from one part of the body to another. Usually, excess energy is directed from painful or over-stimulated areas to those areas needing energy. The first number in the sequence stimulates the area of the body where excess energy has collected and needs to be dissipated; the second number stimulates the area where the excess energy is to be sent to[15].

Other Mandarin Chinese healing sounds and words used for healing are listed in Table 7. (See also Table 5, *Healing Sounds for the Organs,* p. 29.)

---

[15] The Lower Dan Tian, located in the lower abdomen, is generally a good place to send excess energy to, as it is the storehouse of the body's energy.

83

Table 7. Healing Sounds Used in Zhi Neng Medicine

Sound	Effect on the Body
wong	stimulates head and brain
ah	stimulates heart and chest
hong	stimulates lower abdomen
woo	stimulates middle abdomen
hah	stimulates lower abdomen
hao	sends a message to the body or the organ to *"Get well!"* (pronounced as *how, hao* means *"Get well!"* in Mandarin)

84

Mind Power

Mind power is creative visualization. You can think yourself well! Thought is often overlooked as a very powerful tool for turning wishes into reality. Just thinking of something gives it *power, energy and life,* so by thinking specific organs and parts of your body well, healthy, strong and whole, you invoke the power of positive thinking. You are sending out messages with your thoughts. You can try to communicate with your subconscious mind to ask your soul for help in restoring your health. Visualize these sick parts glowing bright, white, clear light and getting well.

The same principle applies to negative thoughts. So do not dwell on your illness. Do not be despondent or entertain thoughts that things are getting worse. By doing so, you give power to such thoughts and your subconscious mind will act on them. Similarly, if you have felt some relief from your condition, do not continually check to see whether the pain has indeed gone.

Zhi Neng uses the image of light as healing energy. Think of white light running through your organs and your body, invigorating, and rejuvenating you. You can use a strong golden yellow light with even better results because gold is the highest healing colour in Zhi Neng medicine. The colour aspect of Five Elements Theory is also used in healing visualizations of Zhi Neng medicine.

Zhi Neng Medicine Healing Number 3396815

Chanting has been used for centuries for various purposes. Some chants have evolved into a sequence of sounds with no discernible meaning but with very powerful messages connected to the universe and higher powers. These are known as mantras. Different religions use mantras and chants to stimulate and develop energy in different parts of the body. Mantras are not only sound, but very special messages with incredible power.

Zhi Neng medicine uses a very powerful mantram for universal healing, as shown in Table 8. Repeating *3396815* out loud in Mandarin Chinese, "*San, san, jiu, liu, ba, yao, wu*" stimulates various internal organs, helps balance and develop energy in the body and sends out a message, all at the same time.

"*San, san, jiu, liu, ba, yao, wu,*" can be repeated slowly, rapidly, quietly or loudly anywhere, anytime. Repeating "*San, san, jiu, liu, ba, yao, wu*" is also the key to higher energy development.

Table 8. Zhi Neng Medicine Healing Number 3396815

Number	Mandarin	Pronunciation	Area Stimulated
3	san	*san*	chest
3	san	*san*	chest
9	jiu	*jū* (like *jew*)	lower abdomen
6	liu	*lū* (like *ewe*)	ribs
8	ba	*bah*	navel
1	yao	*yow* (like *cow*)	head
5	wu	*woo*	stomach

Sha's Golden Healing Ball

The geometry of the sphere is very powerful in nature. The earth can be seen as a ball, the planets are balls, the sun is a glowing ball. You can see roundness in everything, in embryos, cells, organs, water droplets, flower buds, pearls, eggs, fruits, nuts and seeds. Almost everything in the universe has roundness and smoothness in its form. Roundness is very important.

Similarly, spinning energy moving in circular or spiral patterns is very powerful. You can see examples of this in nature and in technology. Atomic particles have their own natural spin, rotation and energy. Planetary motions are elliptical. The earth and other planets in our solar system spin on their axes as they orbit around the sun. Moons move in the same way as they orbit around planets. Matter spinning at high speeds has acceleration and very intense energy. Think of the energy in a tornado or a high-speed engine.

In Eastern philosophies, the concepts of *wu chi* (nothing) and *tai chi* (something) can be symbolized as circles in the Zhi Neng medicine logo (Figure 4). Circles have no end. Balls have no orientation; top becomes bottom becomes top. So too, Yin/Yang is interchangeable and interrelated, as are *wu chi* and *tai chi*. Everything in the universe can be said to be in a state of *wu chi* transforming into *tai chi* (nothing transforms into something), and *tai chi* transforming back into *wu chi* (something transforms into nothing). Taoists understand *wu chi* to be *wu we* (to do nothing); and *tai chi* to be *you wei* (to do something). Buddhists think of *wu chi* as *ding li* (emptiness and nothingness), and *tai chi* as *hui li* (intelligence and stability).

Figure 4. Zhi Neng Medicine Logo

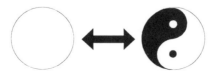

(Wu chi is the empty state.)

This concept of *wu chi* ⇔ *tai chi* interchange can be applied to health. The human body and the internal organs all follow the law of *wu chi* going to *tai chi* and vice versa. Some internal organs can be in the *wu chi* condition, some in the *tai chi* condition. Everything in the body is always in a state of flux, moving constantly between a condition of balance and imbalance. Inflammation in any part of the body is considered to be a *tai chi* condition. If the inflammation clears up, that part goes back to the *wu chi* condition. For example, a healthy stomach is in the *wu chi* condition. If the stomach develops ulcers, *wu chi* has been transformed into *tai chi*.

87

Zhi Neng medicine uses all these principles in the healing technique called *Sha's Golden Healing Ball*. Use your mind to visualize a *spinning golden ball of light* in any part of your body that needs energy or healing. *Why?* Light is energy. Light has healing power. Gold light has the highest healing power of all the colours and lights. Spinning the ball connects it with the energy of the universe. Spinning it faster harnesses more energy.

Visualizing a ball of spinning golden light in your body stimulates and excites the cells in that area. They start vibrating faster and radiate more energy. The increased energy makes the ball spin faster and glow even brighter. It becomes more powerful and generates even more energy. Your cells react to the increased intensity of the ball's field by vibrating even faster and radiating more energy.

The intensity of the ball's field fluctuates constantly as it spins; the energy in the field also changes constantly. This affects the fields of your cells and organs, creating multiple inter-penetrating fields. Energy in the fields with higher intensities will flow to fields of lower intensities and patterns. Energy will collectively flow between tissue groups and organs. Proper energy flow in the body is the first step to good health.

Sha's Golden Healing Ball works by strengthening weak organs, dissipating blocked and excess energy, and balancing energy flow throughout the body. You can play with and spin the ball in any part of your body, for as long as you want, anywhere and anytime, for better health.

If excess energy accumulates and becomes blocked in the body, it may cause pain, fever, inflammation, tumours, cysts or cancer. Visualizing *Sha's Golden Healing Ball* as a golden ball of light, spinning very fast in that area of the body, highly stimulates the cells in the area, making them vibrate much faster. The spinning ball liberates tremendous amounts of energy which are passed on and dissipated through other parts of the body, relieving the energy blockage.

Weakness and fatigue, if not due to cancer or inflammation, occur when there is not enough energy in areas of the body. Strengthen those parts by visualizing a spinning ball of golden light there. Spin it faster! Cells will become highly stimulated and radiate more energy. The intensity of their fields increases and the increased energy is passed on, strengthening other cells and organs. You will start feeling stronger. Weakness and fatigue will lift.

If your heart is weak, visualize and spin the ball in the heart area as fast as you can. *WHOoooosh!!!* If your kidneys are weak, spin the ball in the kidney area. If the arm is weak, spin and turn the ball in the area of the arm. Spin the ball in any part of your body that needs strengthening.

Sha's Golden Healing Ball can also be used for developing and balancing energy in the body, increasing your intelligence, prolonging and improving the quality of your life. Think of a spinning golden ball in any one of the five key energy centres, or imagine one big ball rolling up and down your whole body. Imagine the ball getting brighter, hotter and very intense. Make it spin faster, faster, faster*!!! WWOooo!! Wwooo!! WWOOooooo!!* As you spin the ball, silently read, "*San, san, jiu, liu, ba, yao, wu (3396815).*" Tell yourself, *"I am strong. I am well. I restore my health. Thank you very much. Thank you."*

Long-Distance Healing

The speed of the thinking mind is faster than the speed of light. Long-distance healing is as fast as thought even though the patient and healer are not in the same room physically. The healer is able to heal over the distance separating them by just thinking of the patient. The healing is as effective as if the patient had been treated in person. Healing is successful even if patient and healer have never met.

Many patients experience relief the first time. Other patients need more treatments before they notice an improvement. Some people cannot be helped. Healers who have developed their mind highly enough will know how much they can help and will tell you if they cannot help.

How well long-distance healing works depends on the healer's mind power, the purity of their soul and their energy. There are many other factors to be considered. The patient's soul and mind may not be co-operating. Inherited factors and the seriousness of the illness can also affect the success of long-distance healing.

One Hand Healing Method

Zhi Neng medicine's *One Hand Healing Technique* is used for dissipating energy from areas where the body is not well.

While pointing one hand at the affected area, visualize it glowing and radiating with clear, bright light. Your brain cells radiate energy, stimulating the affected area. This makes the cells in that area vibrate much more. Energy will start radiating out and dissipate in the surrounding tissues. Energy flows, the energy blockage is removed; health is restored.

Steps for the *One Hand Healing Technique* are summarized below:

a) Relax in any comfortable position.
b) Point your hand at the affected area, holding it 12"-20" (30-50 cm) away.
c) Visualize *bright light* radiating in the sick area.
d) Visualize the area as transparent and healthy.
e) Practice 3-5 minutes each time.
f) Practice 3-5 times per day.
g) During healing, continue repeating the Zhi Neng Medicine healing mantra "*San, san, jiu, liu, ba, yao, wu (3396815).*"

Note: Alternate hands for pointing as they tire.

One Hand Near, One Hand Far Healing Method

The method of energy balancing called *One Hand Near, One Hand Far* is based on the field theory of physics. Generally, the *near hand* is placed near the area of the body that is ailing, and the *far hand* is placed further from the body, creating a difference in field intensities. This technique can be used for healing yourself and healing other people.

The placement of the two hands at different distances from the body forms two fields of different intensities between the hands and body surfaces. The hand nearer the body *(near hand)* has a higher-intensity field between it and the body surface it faces than the hand farther away from the body *(far hand)*. Energy will flow from the higher-intensity field to the lower-intensity field. Making energy flow will relieve highly accumulated energy. In turn, this will relieve pain, stiffness, inflammation, and stress in over-excited organs. Energy balance and health are restored when energy flows freely throughout the body.

The *near hand* is placed 4"-8" (10-20 cm) from the body. The hand position to use depends on the ailment being treated. Pointing one finger or all the fingers of the hand to the area of pain or illness is used for dissipating more concentrated energy from that area. Otherwise, the palm of the *near hand* normally faces the area being treated. There is greater energy density in the space between the *near hand* and the body. Energy flows from this part of the body to the part of the body facing the *far hand*.

The *far hand* is placed 12"-20" (30-50 cm) from the body. The palm faces an area that needs energy or the area where energy will be sent. There is a lower-intensity field in the space between the *far hand* and the part of the body it faces. This part of the body receives energy from the part of the body facing the *near hand*.

For example, if one side of the body is hurting, you can simply direct energy from that side to the other side. You can also direct the excess energy from an area to the *Lower Dan Tian,* which is the storehouse of the body's foundation energy. If you have pain in one area and weakness in another, you can put the *near hand* over the painful area and the *far hand* over the place where you need the energy. This helps to relieve the conditions of excess energy and insufficient energy at the same time.

The *One Hand Near, One Hand Far Healing Method* simultaneously uses sound energy, creative visualization and hand positions in its application. Hand positions set up fields of different intensities around the body. Energy in the fields naturally starts flowing from the higher-intensity field to the lower one. Saying various healing sounds out loud or silently stimulates cell vibration in the affected organs and increases the intensity of their fields. In turn, this increases the strength of the fields between the hands and the body part they face, so that more energy flows. Even more energy can be made to flow when you use your brain to imagine a bright path of white light flowing from the part of the body facing the *near hand* to that facing the *far hand*.

The application of this healing technique is discussed using the example of a headache. Zhi Neng medicine considers that there is more energy radiating from the brain tissues than can be quickly dissipated. Energy builds up, and a headache results when there is too much energy in the head.

A safe place to direct this excess energy is to the *Lower Dan Tian.* The palm of the *near hand* faces the headache area and the palm of the *far hand* faces the lower abdomen. This creates a field of higher intensity (greater energy density) in the area of the *near hand* facing the head, and a field of lower intensity (lower energy density) in the area of the *far hand* facing the lower abdomen.

The number for head is *1* or *yi;* the number for the lower abdomen is *9* or *jiu.* The number combination for transferring headache energy to the lower abdomen is *1-9* or *yi-jiu.* Repeat the numbers out loud or silently to stimulate energy transfer: *yi-jiu, yi-jiu, yi-jiu, yi-jiu, yi-jiu….*

At the same time, visualize a path of white light flowing from the area of the headache to the lower abdomen. *Energy will flow.* Do this three to five minutes per time and three to five times a day depending on the severity of the headache.

93

Summary of Procedure

The key points to remember in using the *One Hand Near, One Hand Far Healing Technique* for any health problem are summarized below:

a) Relax the body in any comfortable position.
b) Both hands face the body. Don't point the hands away from the body (unless otherwise noted).
c) Place the *near hand* 4"-8" (10-20 cm) from the body. The palm faces the body or the finger(s) point at a body part.
d) Place the *far hand* 12"-20" (30-50 cm) from the body. The palm faces the body or the finger(s) point at a body part.
e) Repeat the healing *sounds* or the healing numbers.
f) *Visualize* bright, glowing light flowing from the body area facing the *near hand* to the body area facing the *far hand*.
g) Practice 3-5 minutes per session.
h) Practice 3-5 times a day.
i) Alternate hands as required or for comfort. However, be careful to observe the correct placement of the *near hand* and the *far hand*.

Healing Methods
for over 100 Common Ailments

Zhi Neng medicine healing techniques for more than 100 common ailments are presented in this section. Health problems are categorized by body and organ location in the *Contents* at the beginning of the book. Refer to Figure 5 for the locations of the various internal organs in the body.

Try these hand-fields healing techniques for three to five minutes at a time, three to five times a day for your health problems. Some problems are helped immediately after only one application.

More serious problems and chronic conditions need time, patience and regular practice before you will notice any results. Many ailments, such as deafness and crossed eyes, are slow to respond. Don't be unreasonable in expecting chronic pain that may have taken years to develop to disappear in a few token treatments. Be patient. Think positively. Apply the healing methods confidently and regularly, and you will see results.

Figure 5.   Basic Anatomy of the Organs

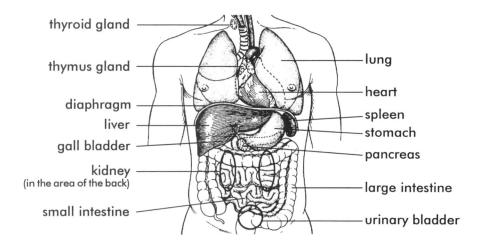

Start Healing Now!

Start using the healing procedures in this section of the book right away if you are in pain or if you have an immediate health concern.

Zhi Neng medicine healing techniques work whether or not you understand or believe in the simple principles of physics that they are based upon. The healing techniques given were all designed to help your body's energy to flow – from areas of high concentration to areas of lower concentration. Healing starts as soon as you put these steps into action!

How To Use this Section

The format used in this section devotes one page to each health condition. Simple instructions are given for the placement of your hands, the sounds to make and the images to visualize. For clarity, refer to the photographs shown for each condition.

The key points of each healing technique are summarized to include the following information:

· **Layman's Description** and/or the medical term for the condition
· **NH:** the *near hand* placement
  (the palm faces the body unless otherwise noted)
· **FH:** the *far hand* placement
  (the palm faces the body unless otherwise noted)
· **Sounds:** the *healing sounds* to use and to say out loud
  (the healing numbers are given, followed by the Mandarin phonetics)
· **Visualize:** the *light* image to visualize and/or the *flow path* for it
· **Notes:** additional information relating to the condition

Remember to be relaxed. Practice earnestly and seriously. Practice 3-5 minutes per application, 3-5 times daily. *Hao! Hao! Hao!*

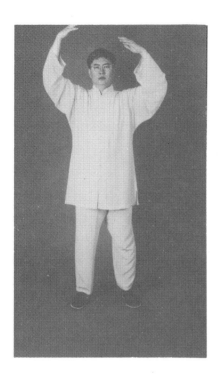

dizziness

NH: side of the head

FH: upper, opposite side of the head

Sound: 1-1, 1-1, *yi-yi, yi-yi*

Visualize: bright, white light glowing in the whole of the brain

Notes: Alternate the hand positions to complete this procedure. This condition is commonly caused by poor capillary circulation in the head.

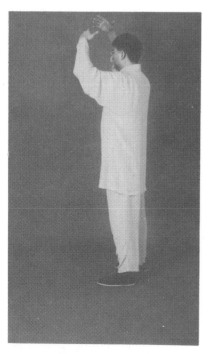

headache, parietal
(crown area)

NH: over the crown of the head

FH: lower abdomen (Lower Dan Tian)

Sound: 1-9, 1-9, *yi-jiu, yi-jiu*

Visualize: light flowing from the crown of the head to the lower abdomen

Notes: This conition is related to liver problems and to the liver (Foot Jue Yin) meridian.

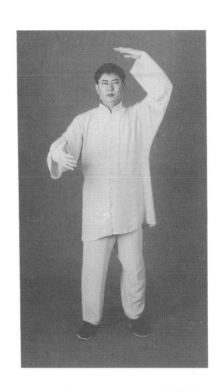

97

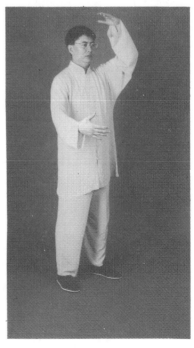

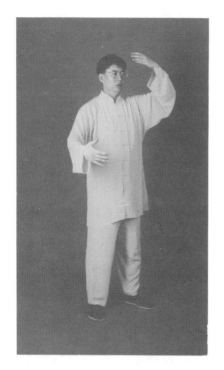

headache, frontal (forehead area)

NH: forehead or facing the point midway between the eyebrows (Yin Tang)

FH: lower abdomen (Lower Dan Tian)

Sound: 1-9, 1-9, *yi-jiu, yi-jiu*

Visualize: light flowing from the forehead to the lower abdomen

Notes: This condition is related to the stomach (Foot Yang Ming) meridian.

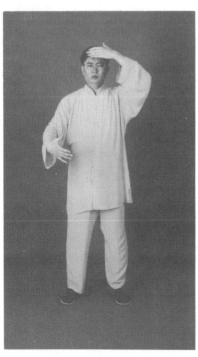

headache, temporal (temple area)

NH: 4 finger tips point downwards towards the temple

FH: lower abdomen (Lower Dan Tian)

Sound: 1-9, 1-9, *yi-jiu, yi-jiu*

Visualize: light flowing from the temple area to the lower abdomen

Notes: Do not point upwards with the near hand. Alternate the hands if there is pain in both temples. This condition is related to the gall bladder meridian.

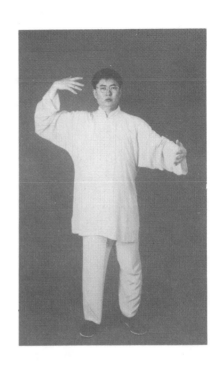

99

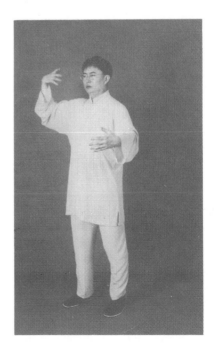

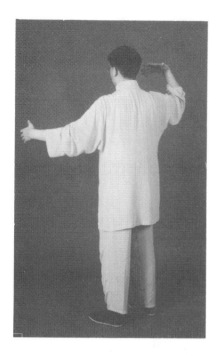

headache, sub-occipital (base of the neck)

NH: 4 finger tips point at the back of the neck

FH: lower abdomen (Lower Dan Tian)

Sound: 1-9, 1-9, *yi-jiu, yi-jiu*

Visualize: light flowing from the back of the head to the lower abdomen

Notes: This condition is commonly caused by tension in the neck.

100

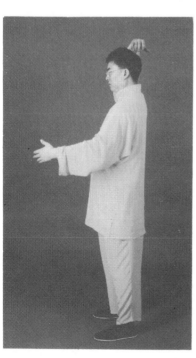

high blood pressure
high systolic, high diastolic
(hypertension I)

NH: over the crown area of the head or facing the forehead

FH: lower abdomen (Lower Dan Tian)

Sound: 1-9, 1-9, *yi-jiu, yi-jiu*

Visualize: light flowing from the head to the lower abdomen

Notes: Use this procedure if the patient has high systolic and high diastolic blood pressure.

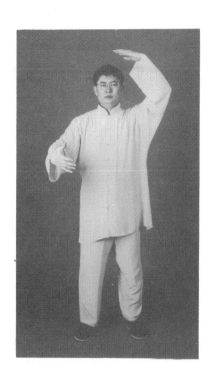

101

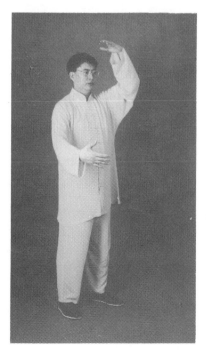

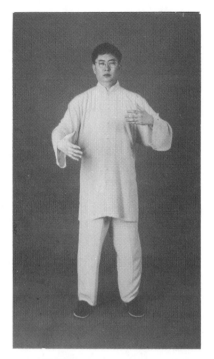

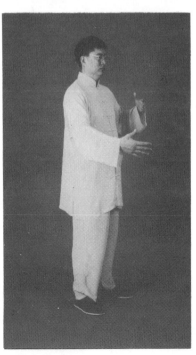

high blood pressure
normal systolic, high diastolic
(hypertension II)

NH: heart, or facing the middle of the chest (Middle Dan Tian)

FH: lower abdomen (Lower Dan Tian)

Sound: 2-9, 2-9, *ar-jiu, ar-jiu*

Visualize: light flowing from the heart to the lower abdomen

Notes: Use this procedure when the patient has normal systolic pressure and high diastolic pressure. This is a condition of too much energy in the heart.

low blood pressure (hypotension)

NH: lower abdomen (Lower Dan Tian)

FH: crown area of the head, the forehead or the point midway between the eyebrows (Yin Tang)

Sound: 9-1, 9-1, *jiu-yi, jiu-yi*

Visualize: light flowing from the lower abdomen to the head

Notes: Do not use this procedure if the patient has glaucoma.

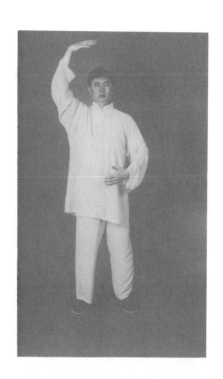

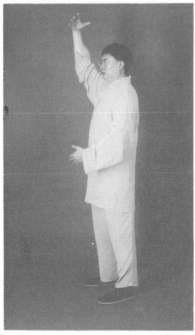

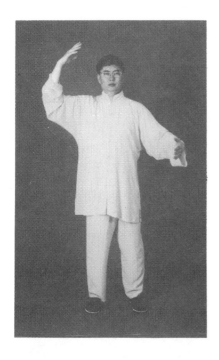

stroke
(left-side paralysis)

NH: right palm faces, or the fingers of the right hand point to the right side of the brain

FH: left hand faces the left side of the body

Sound: 1-9, 1-9, *yi-jiu, yi-jiu*

Visualize: light flowing from the right side of the head to the left side of the body

Notes: Paralysis on the left side of the body is due to a hemorrhage or a blood clot (energy blockage) on the right side of the brain.

Take care to position the near hand and the far hand correctly; reversing the hand positions may worsen the condition!

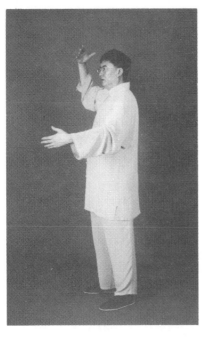

stroke
(right-side paralysis)

NH: left side of the head

FH: right side of the body

Sound: 1-9, 1-9 *yi-jiu, yi-jiu*

Visualize: light flowing from the left side of the head to the right side of the body

Notes: Paralysis of the right side of the body is due to hemorrhage or ruptured blood vessels on the left side of the brain.

Take care to position the near hand and the far hand correctly; reversing the hand positions may worsen the condition!

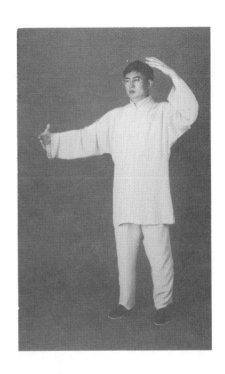

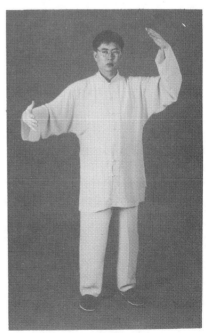

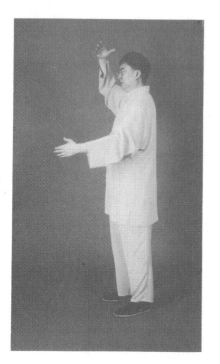

hardening of the arteries in the brain (cerebral arteriosclerosis)

NH: any side of the head; shake the hand rapidly

FH: lower abdomen (Lower Dan Tian)

Sound: 1-9, 1-9, *yi-jiu, yi-jiu*

Visualize: light flowing from the head to the lower abdomen or visualize bright light spreading throughout the brain

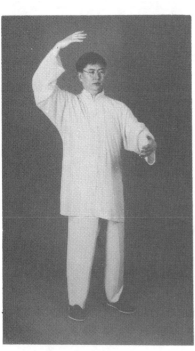

brain tumour

NH: shake and point the middle finger at the tumour at a distance of 5 cm

FH: lower abdomen (Lower Dan Tian)

Sound: 1-9, 1-9, *yi-jiu, yi-jiu*

Visualize: light flowing from the head to the lower abdomen or visualize light spreading out and dissipating from the area of the tumour

Notes: Don't think about the tumour. Instead, think that the affected area is healthy and glowing with light.

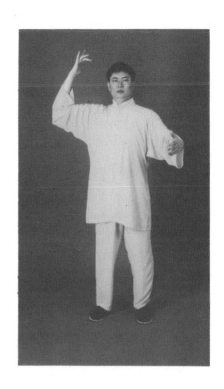

107

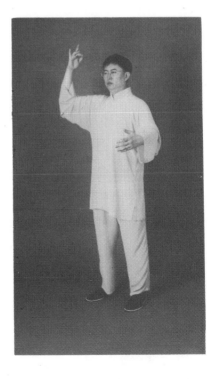

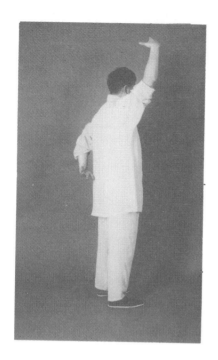

senility, dementia, Alzheimer's Disease

NH: kidney area in the lower back or the Snow Mountain Area

FH: over the crown area of the head

Sound: 9-1, 9-1, jiu-yi, jiu-yi

Visualize: light flowing from the Snow Mountain Area up the spinal column to the Bai Hui acupuncture point and nourishing the brain

Notes: Do not use this method if the patient has high blood pressure.

hyperactivity
(in children)

One Hand Method: pat the child's head or shake one hand 5 cm over the crown of the child's head

Sound: 1-1, 1-1, *yi-yi, yi-yi*

Visualize: bright light from the universe flowing into the child's brain

Notes: When performing this healing procedure, visualize and think of the child as being smart and intelligent.

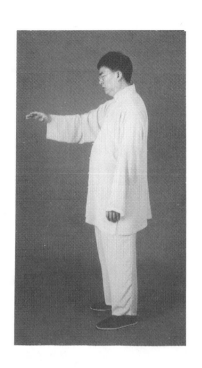

109

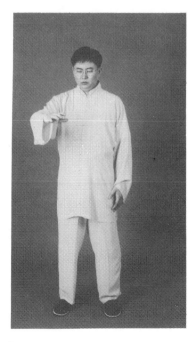

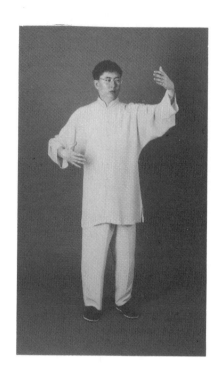

nearsightedness (recent onset)

NH: right palm diagonally at the liver, and shaking

FH: forehead or the point midway between the eyebrows (Yin Tang); if the liver condition is weak, the far hand faces the lower abdomen

Sound: 7-1, 7-1, *chi-yi, chi-yi*

Visualize: light flowing from the liver to the Yin Tang point

Notes: "The liver opens on the eyes." In traditional Chinese medicine, the eye is connected with the liver meridian; the eyes often reflects the health of the liver.

cataracts

One Hand Method: cup the finger tips (as if holding an eyeball) at a distance ~5 cm from the eye

Sound: 1-1, 1-1, *yi-yi, yi-yi*

Visualize: bright light dissipating from the eye; imagine the surface-layer cells of the eyeball vibrating; see the eyeball as being clean, shiny and clear

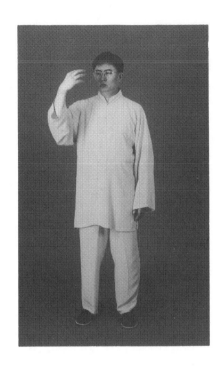

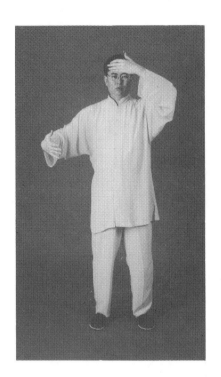

glaucoma

NH: forehead or the point midway between the eyebrows (Yin Tang)

FH: palm facing the liver diagonally

Sound: 1-7, 1-7, *yi-chi, yi-chi*

Visualize: light flowing from the Yin Tang point to the liver

Notes: Do not point the *near hand* directly at the eye as too much energy can harm the delicate tissues of the eye.

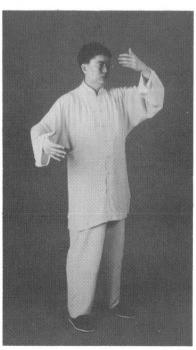

retinal atrophy

NH: centre of the lower back (Ming Men point)

FH: forehead or the midpoint between the eyebrows (Yin Tang)

Sound: 9-1, 9-1, *jiu-yi, jiu-yi*

Visualize: light flowing from the lower back (Snow Mountain Area) or from the lower abdomen (Lower Dan Tian) to the Yin Tang point

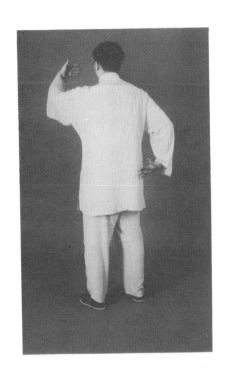

113

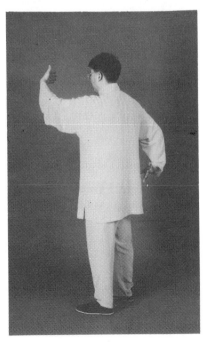

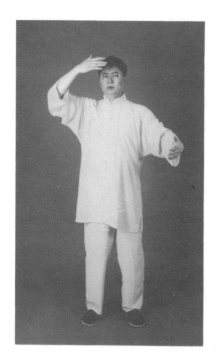

styes and sore, irritated eyes (opthalmia, conjunctivitis)

NH: forehead or midpoint between the eyebrows (Yin Tang)

FH: lower abdomen (Lower Dan Tian)

Sound: 1-9, 1-9, *yi-jui, yi-jui*

Visualize: light flowing from the Yin Tang point to the Lower Dan Tian

114

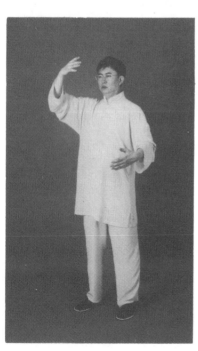

chronic tearing (dacryocystitis)

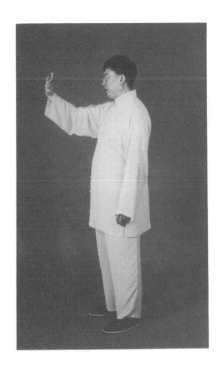

One Hand Method: hold the palm steady at a distance of ~30 cm from the affected eye(s)

Sound: 1-1, 1-1, *yi-yi, yi-yi*

Visualize: none; just stare at the palm of your hand; use both eyes to stare at the palm without blinking – this forces the eyes to start watering and tearing

Notes: Chronic tearing is the result of blocked tear ducts. Forcing the eyes not to blink will stimulate tear production. This action helps to cleanse and remove blockages from the tear ducts.

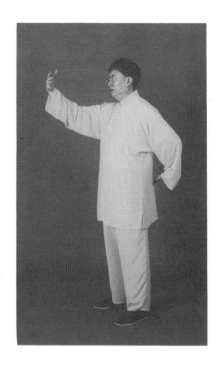

seeing spots or lines in front of the eye (floaters)

NH: lower abdomen (Lower Dan Tian) or the lower back / kidney area (Snow Mountain Area)

FH: eyes

Sound: 9-1, 9-1, *jiu-yi, jiu-yi*

Visualize: light flowing from the kidney area (Snow Mountain Area) to the point midway between the eyebrows (Yin Tang)

Notes: If the kidney is weak, develop more kidney energy first (practice the healing technique for **Kidney Inflammation,** see page 160).

crossed eyes (strabismus)

Hands: put the backs of both hands together, and gradually pull them apart in front of your eyes

Sound: 1-1, 1-1, *yi-yi, yi-yi*

Visualize: the eyes separating or aligning properly

Notes: This condition takes time to recover from and needs to be repeated many times. Move one hand if only one eye is crossed, moving the hand as if aligning the eye. For **walled eyes** (the opposite of crossed eyes), start with the backs of the hands eye-width apart and slowly bring them together.

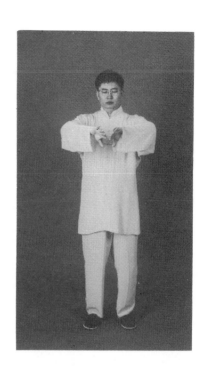

117

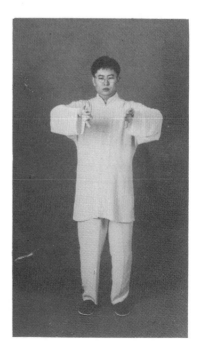

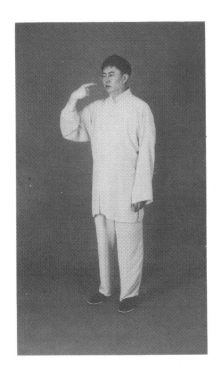

congestion in one nostril (nasal sinusitis and rhinitis)

STEP 1

One Hand Method: shake your hand at the blocked nostril

Sound: 2-2, *ar-ar* or 3-5, *san-wu*

Visualize: bright light spreading out from the blocked nostril

STEP 2

One Hand Method: point the index finger at a distance of ~5 cm from the blocked nostril or the point midway between the eyebrows (Yin Tang acupuncture point)

Sound: 1-3-5, *1-3-5, yi san-wu, yi-san-wu*

Visualize: light flowing from the nostril, through the lungs and the stomach into the Lower Dan Tian (lower abdomen)

congestion in both nostrils (chronic nasal sinusitis and rhinitis)

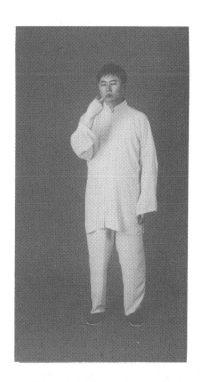

STEP 1

NH: spread the index and the middle fingers in a **V** at both nostrils

FH: lower abdomen (Lower Dan Tian); shake the hand

Sound: 2-2, 2-2, *ar-ar, ar-ar*

Visualize: light glowing in the nose

STEP 2

NH: point the index and the middle fingers ~5 cm from both sides of the Yin Tang (the midpoint between the eyebrows); the fingers point downwards slightly

FH: stomach

Sound: 1-3-5, *1-3-5, yi san-wu, yi-san-wu*

Visualize: light flowing from the nose to the stomach

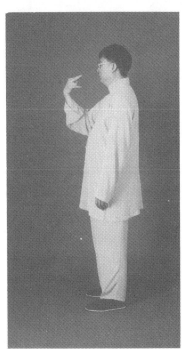

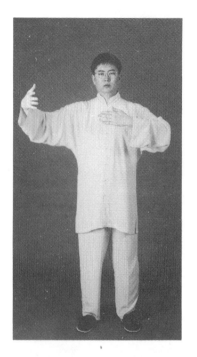

120

stuffy or runny nose (due to colds, allergies or inflammation)

NH: middle of the chest, above the level of the nipples

FH: side of the body, at chest level

Sound: 3-5, 3-5, *san-wu, san-wu*

Visualize: light flowing from the nose down to the stomach

Notes: This is a condition of energy not flowing properly in the lungs.

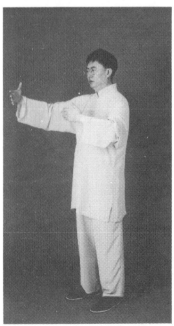

stuffy nose and sinuses with fever
(acute rhinitis and sinusitis)

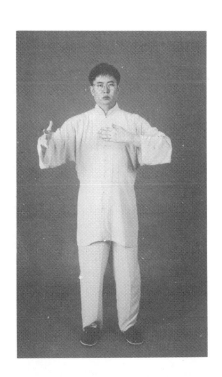

NH: chest area

FH: extend the arm (at chest level) with the fingers pointing straight ahead and away from the body

Sound: 3-5, 3-5, *san-wu, san-wu*

Visualize: light flowing from the lungs to the stomach

Notes: Do for 2 minutes only. Do not practice this technique too long because the fingers are pointing out and directing energy away from the body.

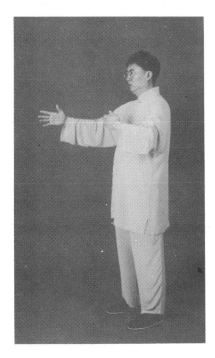

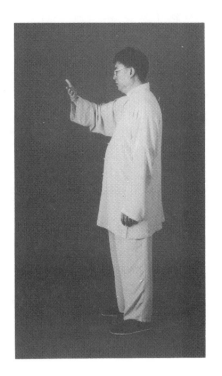

chronic post-nasal drip

One Hand Method: the palm is tilted up slightly, facing the nose area or midpoint between the eyebrows (the Yin Tang acupuncture point)

Sound: 3-1, 3-1, *san-yi, san-yi*

Visualize: light flowing from the lungs to the nose

Conditions of the Mouth

cold sores or cankers that form cavities (Herpes Simplex I)

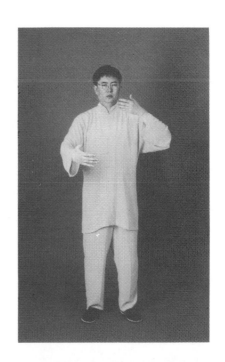

NH: middle finger points to the canker

FH: stomach; the hand angled slightly downwards

Sound: 1-5-9, *yi-wu-jiu*

Visualize: light flowing from the canker, through the stomach and into the lower abdomen

Notes: Use this technique for treating cold sores or cankers that form cavities (internal deprssions) around the lips or inside the mouth.

123

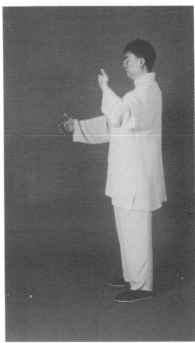

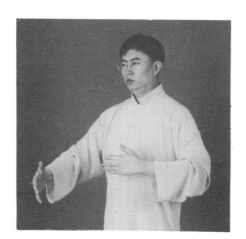

cold sores or cankers that form protrusions (Herpes Simplex II)

NH: stomach

FH: lower abdomen

Sound: 5-9, 5-9, *wu-jiu, wu-jiu*

Visualize: light flowing from the canker, through the stomach and into the lower abdomen

Notes: Use this technique for cold sores and cankers that form external blisters or mound-like protrusions in and around the mouth.

enlarged tongue

NH: right palm, face up, above navel

FH: left palm, face up, below navel

Sound: 3-3-9-6-8-1-5, *san-san-jiu-liu-ba-yao-wu*

Visualize: the numbers 3-3-9-6-8-1-5

Notes: Teeth indentations along the edges of the tongue indicates weak Qi energy.

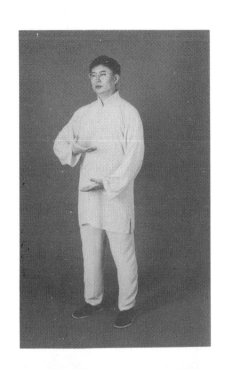

125

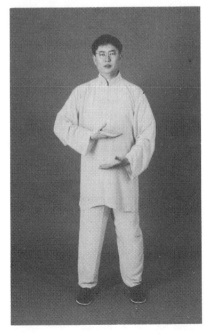

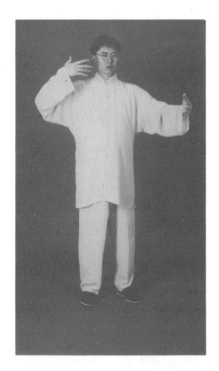

toothache, swollen gums (gingivitis)

NH: four fingers point to the affected area

FH: upper abdomen, the stomach

Sound: 1-5-9, 1-5-9, *yi-wu-jiu, yi-wu-jiu*

Visualize: light flowing from the affected area to the lower abdomen

Notes: Swollen gums are a sign of too much energy in the stomach.

126

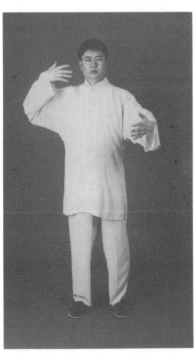

receding gums, periodontal disease

NH: lower abdomen (Lower Dan Tian)

FH: mouth and gums

Sound: 9-1, 9-1, *jiu-yi, jiu-yi,*

Visualize: light flowing from the lower abdomen to the affected area

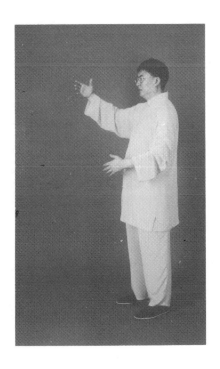

127

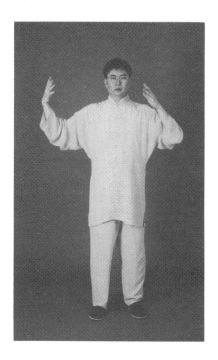

facial paralysis
with mouth twisted to the left
(Bell's Palsy I)

NH: left side of the face (the twisted side)

FH: right side of the face (the smooth side)

Sound: 1-1, 1-1, *yi-yi, yi-yi*

Visualize: light flowing from the left (twisted) side of the face to the right (smooth) side of the face

Notes: Left side disfigurement of the mouth is due to paralysis of the facial nerve on the right side of the face. The smooth side is the weak side – the muscles are weak; so send energy to the weak side.

facial paralysis
with mouth twisted to the right
(Bell's Palsy II)

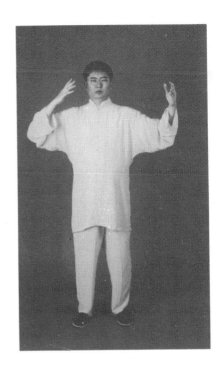

NH: right side of the face (the twisted side)

FH: left side of the face (the smooth side)

Sound: 1-1, 1-1, *yi-yi, yi-yi*

Visualize: light flowing from the right (twisted) side of the face to the left (smooth) side of the face

Notes: Right side disfigurement of the mouth is due to paralysis of the facial nerve on the left side of the face. The smooth side is the weak side – the muscles are weak; so send energy to the weak side.

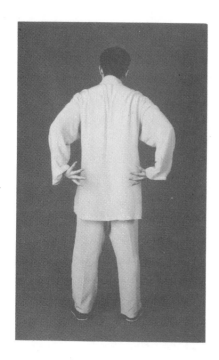

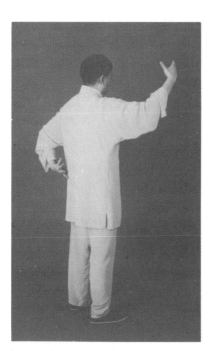

ringing in the ears (tinnitus)

STEP 1

NH: the lower back (Snow Mountain Area)

FH: the lower back (Snow Mountain Area)

Sound: 9-9, 9-9, jiu-jiu, jiu-jiu

Visualize: bright light building up in the lower back and in the kidneys

STEP 2

NH: kidney area

FH: affected ear

Sound: 9-1, 9-1, jiu-yi, jiu-yi

Visualize: bright light flowing from the kidney to the affected ear

Notes: This is a situation where the kidney Qi is weak. Standard treatment would include Qi Gong, herbs and acupuncture. Treatment may take months for chronic or long-term conditions.

deafness

NH: affected ear

FH: opposite ear

Sound: 1-1, 1-1, *yi-yi, yi-yi*

Visualize: light flowing from the affected ear to the other ear

Notes: Alternate hand positions if both ears are affected.

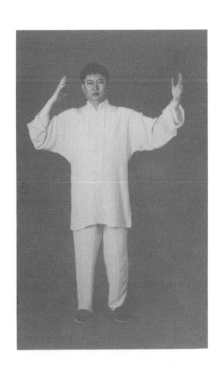

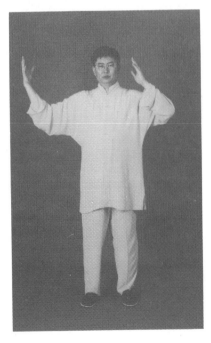

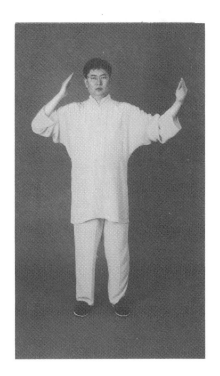

hearing loss
(hearing that is not clear)

NH: cup the affected ear (do not touch)

FH: palm faces the opposite ear

Sound: 1-1, 1-1, *yi-yi, yi-yi*

Visualize: light flowing from the affected ear to the other ear

Notes: Alternate hands if both ears are affected. Be persistent as this is a slow process.

deafness caused by drugs (iatrogenic deafness)

NH: affected ear

FH: opposite ear

Sound: 1-1, 1-1, *yi-yi, yi-yi*

Visualize: light flowing from the affected ear to the other ear

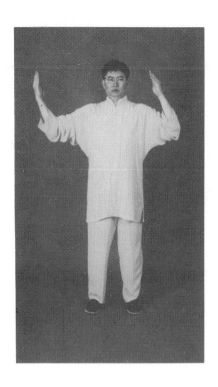

133

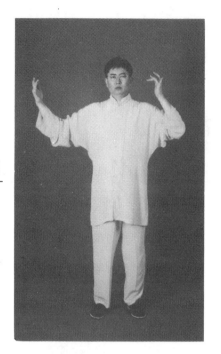

earache due to middle ear inflammation (otitis media)

NH: middle finger points at the affected ear

FH: lower abdomen (Lower Dan Tian)

Sound: 1-9, 1-9, *yi-jiu, yi-jiu*

Visualize: light flowing from the affected ear to the lower abdomen

Notes: Refer to the upper photo (the *far hand* placement should be lower than that shown). This procedure is more effective than the **Alternative Method** described below.

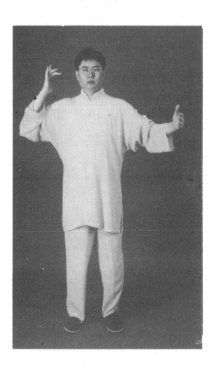

ALTERNATIVE METHOD (one ear good)

NH: middle finger points to the affected ear

FH: palm faces the good ear

Sound: 1-1, 1-1, *yi-yi, yi-yi*

Visualize: light flowing from the affected ear to the good ear

Notes: Refer to the lower photo.

Conditions of the Neck

chronic sore throat (pharyngitis, tonsillitis, laryngitis)

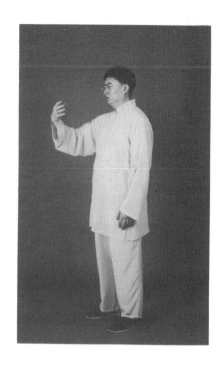

One Hand Method: point the finger tips and the thumb towards the throat, opening and closing them continuously

Sound: 1-1, 1-1, *yi-yi, yi-yi*

Visualize: the membranes of the throat stretching, and becoming smooth and elastic

Notes: Hoarseness of voice, chronic throat inflammations, and throat membranes that feel rough and tight are symptoms all related to the Middle Dan Tian. Consult a medical doctor if the condition lasts for more than 4-6 weeks as it may be indicative of a more serious problem.

135

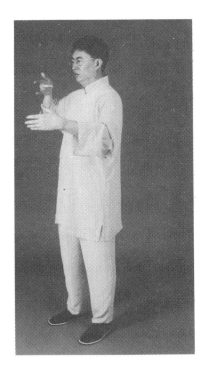

acute throat inflammation (strep throat)

NH: middle finger points to the throat

FH: lower abdomen (Lower Dan Tian)

Sound: 1-9, 1-9, *yi-jiu, yi-jiu*

Visualize: light flowing from the throat area to the lower abdomen

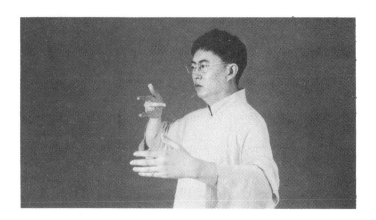

mumps
(swollen facial or parotid glands)

NH: stomach

FH: lungs; hands pointed slightly outwards (to reduce the energy of the stomach)

Sound: 5-3, 5-3, *wu-san, wu-san*

Visualize: light dissipating from the lungs

Notes: Do for 3 minutes only.
This condition is due to excessive energy in the lungs and in the stomach. Do not eat cold foods like ice-cream or drink ice drinks.

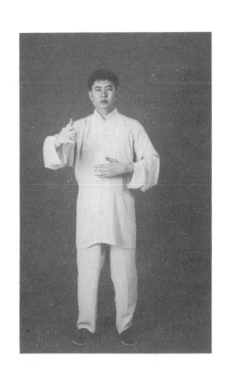

137

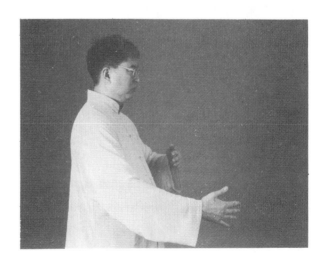

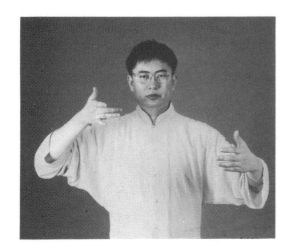

thyroid tumour

NH: middle finger points to the thyroid tumour

FH: right auricle of the heart

Sound: 1-2, 1-2, *yi-ar, yi-ar*

Visualize: light flowing and dissipating from the area of the tumour

thyroid gland
(hyperthyroidism)

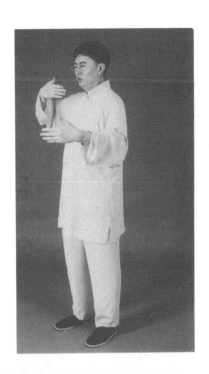

NH: middle finger points to the thyroid gland

FH: right auricle of the heart

Sound: 1-2, 1-2, *yi-ar, yi-ar*

Visualize: light flowing from the thyroid gland to the right auricle of the heart

Notes: Narrow veins returning to the right auricle are often a congenital condition.

139

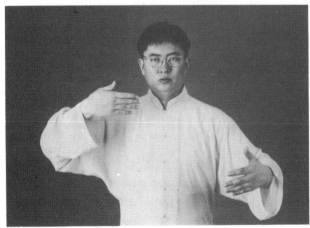

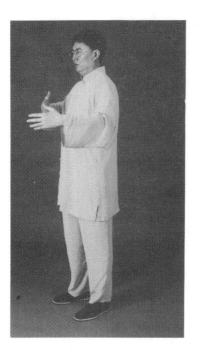

bronchitis, tracheitis, asthma, pulmonary emphysema

NH: affected lung

FH: opposite lung

Sound: 3-3, 3-3, *san-san, san-san*

Visualize: light dissipating from the affected lung

Notes: Alternate hands if both lungs are affected.

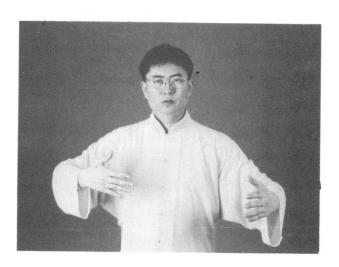

tuberculosis

STEP 1 OF 2

NH: kidney area

FH: lower back (Snow Mountain Area)

Sound: 9-9, *jiu-jiu or hong-hong*

Visualize: both kidneys glowing with light

Notes: This condition is typically due to exhaustion of Yin energy. Step 1 is performed first to build up energy in the kidney area.

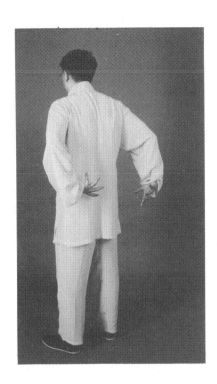

141

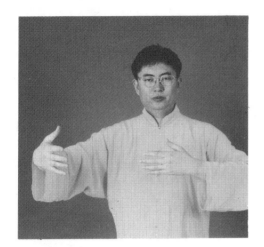

tuberculosis

STEP 2 OF 2

NH: lungs

FH: the side of the body

Sound: 2-2, *ar, ar* or 3-3, *san-san*

Visualize: light dissipating from the lungs

Notes: Alternate the hands.

excess phlegm

NH: at the center of the chest

FH: at the side of the chest

Sound: 2-2, *ar, ar* or 3-3, *san-san*

Visualize: light dissipating from the chest

Notes: This condition is due to excess lung energy.

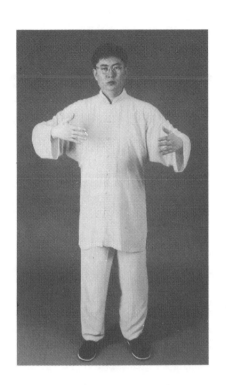

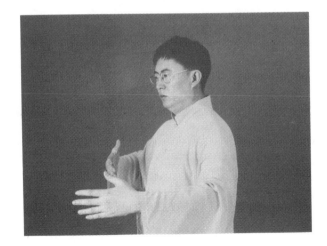

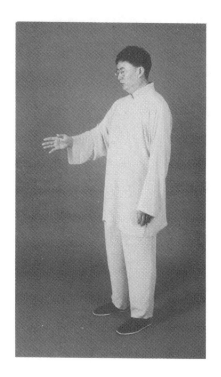

whooping cough (pertussis)

One Hand Method: palm faces the stomach

Sound: 5-9, 5-9, *wu-jiu, wu-jiu*

Visualize: the stomach glowing bright light and getting well

Conditions of the Heart

heart
(all heart conditions)

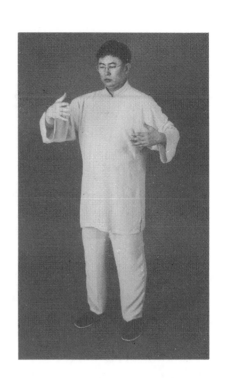

NH: left side of heart at left nipple

FH: right side of left nipple, a little higher than the *near hand*

Sound: 2-2, 2-2, *ar-ar, ar-ar*

Visualize: the whole heart healthy and glowing with light

145

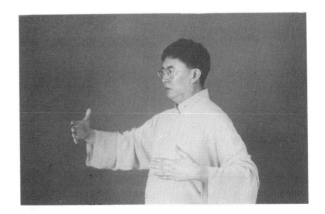

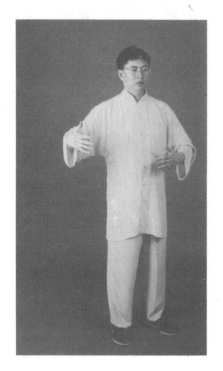

stomach inflammation &/or enlarged liver

STEP 1 OF 2
(see pages 147-8 for STEP 2)

NH: Left hand faces the stomach

FH: right hand faces the liver

Sound: 5-7, 5-7, *wu-chi, wu-chi*

Visualize: light flowing from the stomach to the liver

Notes: After 2 minutes of Step 1, continue with Step 2 as described below. This treatment facilitates portal vein drainage.

This is Step 1 of 2 for the conditions of:

a) **Stomach Inflammation** or gastritis (see page 147 for Step 2)

b) **Enlarged Liver**, symptomized by a bloated feeling in the liver (see page 148 for Step 2)

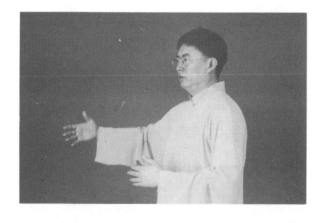

stomach inflammation, gastritis

STEP 2 OF 2
(see page 146 for STEP 1)

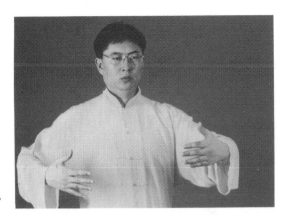

NH: right hand shakes and points at the liver

FH: right auricle of the heart, on the right side of the left nipple

Sound: 7-2, 7-2, *chi-ar, chi-ar*

Visualize: light flowing from the liver to the right auricle

Notes: Stop after 2 minutes. Repeat both steps.

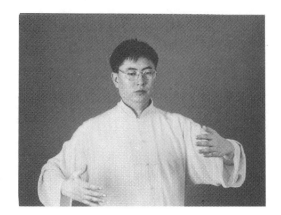

enlarged liver, bloated feeling in the liver

STEP 2 OF 2
(see page 146 for STEP 1)

NH: liver

FH: center of the chest (Middle Dan Tian)

Sound: 7-2, 7-2, *chi-ar, chi-ar*

Visualize: light flowing from the liver area to the right auricle of the heart

Notes: Stop after 2 minutes. Repeat both steps.

duodenal ulcer

NH: stomach

FH: lower abdomen (Lower Dan Tian)

Sound: 5-9, 5-9, *wu-jiu, wu-jiu*

Visualize: light dissipating from the stomach area

Notes: Do for 3 minutes maximum only; practicing too long may cause *descended stomach.*

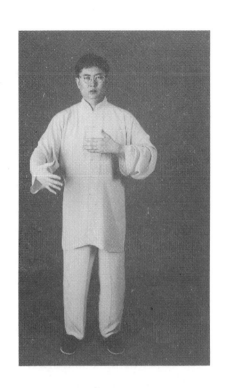

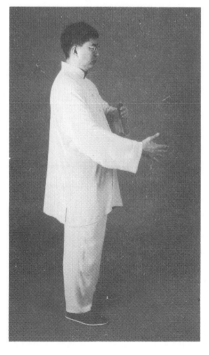

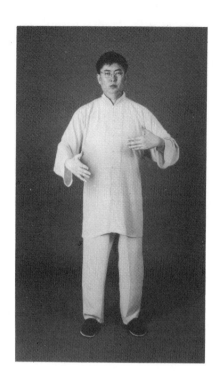

descended stomach

NH: below the stomach, the palm angled slightly upwards

FH: upper abdomen

Sound: 9-5, 9-5, *jiu-wu, jiu-wu*

Visualize: the stomach being raised up

enlarged spleen (splenomegaly)

STEP 1 OF 3

NH: spleen

FH: liver

Sound: 7-7, *chi-chi*

Visualize: light flowing from the spleen to the liver

Notes: Do for 2-3 minutes only. Proceed with Step 2.

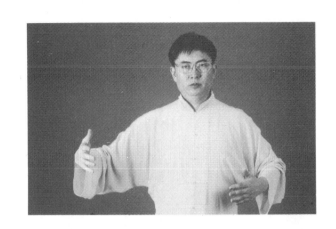

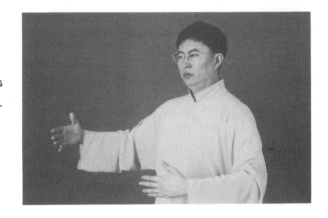

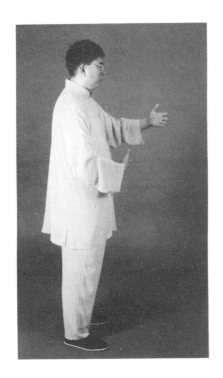

enlarged spleen (splenomegaly)

STEP 2 OF 3

NH: liver

FH: center of the chest, above the level of the nipples

Sound: 7-2, 7-2, *chi-ar, chi-ar*

Visualize: light flowing from the liver to the right auricle (at the right side of heart)

Notes: Do for 2-3 minutes only. Proceed with Step 3.

enlarged spleen (splenomegaly)

STEP 3 OF 3

NH: left side of the heart, at nipple level (left side of of left nipple)

FH: right side of the heart, at nipple level

Sound: 2-2, 2-2, *ar-ar, ar-ar*

Visualize: the whole heart being healthy and glowing with a bright red light

Notes: Perform this last step for 5 minutes.

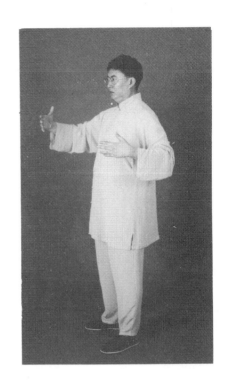

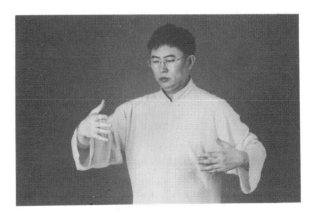

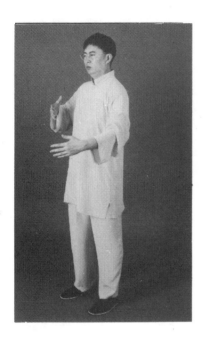

diabetes

NH: pancreas or 1" above pancreas (left front stomach area)

FH: palm angled up (slightly) towards the bladder and facing the lower abdomen (Lower Dan Tian)

Sound: 5-9, 5-9, *wu-jiu, wu-jiu*

Visualize: light flowing from the pancreas to the lower abdomen

Notes: Do for 3 minutes only. Diabetes is a condition where the pancreas is not producing enough insulin; there is excess energy in the pancreas. Patients usually experience excessive thirst and excessive urination.

Conditions in the Liver and Gall Bladder

liver inflammation

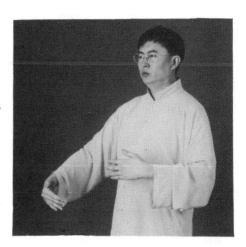

NH: palm faces the liver or the fingers point towards the liver

FH: lower abdomen (Lower Dan Tian)

Sound: 7-9, 7-9, chi-jiu, chi-jiu

Visualize: light flowing from the liver to the lower abdomen

155

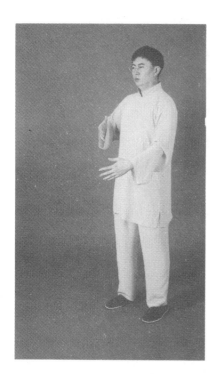

jaundice
(caused by hepatitis)

NH: right hand faces the liver

FH: left hand faces the urinary bladder area, pointing slightly downwards

Sound: 7-9, 7-9, *chi-jiu, chi-jiu*

Visualize: light flowing from the liver to the lower abdomen

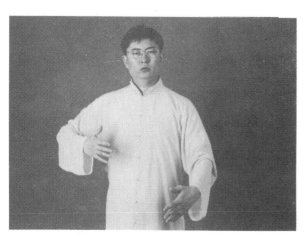

cirrhosis of the liver

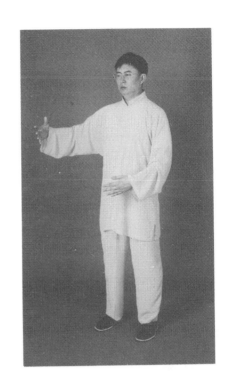

STEP 1

NH: lower abdomen (Lower Dan Tian)

FH: liver
(right front, rib area)

Sound: 9-7, 9-7, jiu-chi, jiu-chi

Visualize: light flowing from the lower abdomen (Lower Dan Tian) to the liver

Notes: Hardening of the liver tissues is due to inadequate cell vibration in the liver cells. The lliver is lacking in Qi energy.

STEP 2

Use the same technique as for Heart Conditions (see page 145).

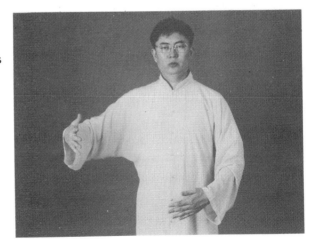

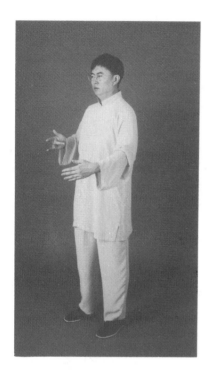

gall stones and gall bladder inflammation (cholecystitis)

STEP 1
(use for inflammation and for gall stones)

NH: middle finger points toward the gall bladder (right front rib area)

FH: lower abdomen (Lower Dan Tian)

Sound: 7-9, 7-9, *chi-jiu, chi-jiu*

Visualize: light radiating from the gall bladder to the lower abdomen (Lower Dan Tian)

Notes: When gall stones move out of the gall bladder, patients will feel severe pain. Use Step 2 at this point.

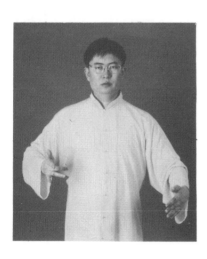

STEP 2
(use for breaking up gall stones)

NH: middle finger points towards the lower abdomen (Lower Dan Tian)

FH: gall bladder area

Sound: 9-7, 9-7, *jiu-chi, jiu-chi*

Visualize: a laser beam of light breaking up the gall stones

Notes: Step 2 is used to transfer energy from the Lower Dan Tian to break up the gall stones.

hepatitis B

NH: facing the liverr, and being shaken

FH: lower abdomen (Lower Dan Tian)

Sound: 7-9, 7-9, *chi-jiu, chi-jiu*

Visualize: light radiating and dissipating from the liver

Notes: Hepatitis B is a condition where there are too few liver cells, and too much energy in these few cells.

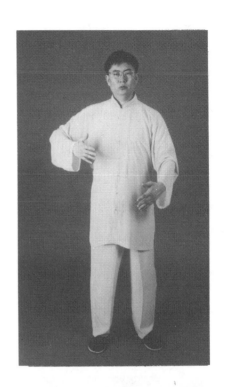

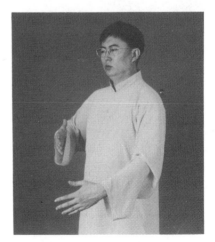

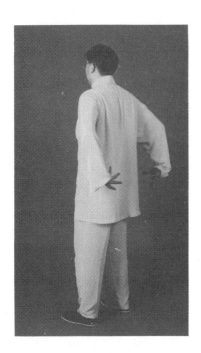

kidney inflammation, kidney atrophy, kidney stones (acute and chronic nephritis)

NH: affected kidney

FH: other kidney or the lower back (Snow Mountain Area)

Sound: 9-9, 9-9, *jiu-jiu, jiu-jiu*

Visualize: light dissipating from the kidney area

Notes: If a kidney stone or a tumour is present, use the middle finger of the *near hand* to point at it. Visualize a laser beam of light emitting from the finger. Aim the laser beam at the tumour or kidney stone to dissolve it.

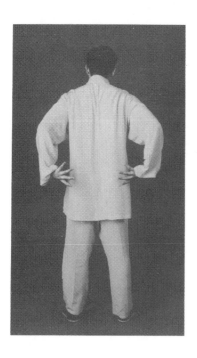

urinary tract inflammation, urinary bladder inflammation (urethritis, cystitis)

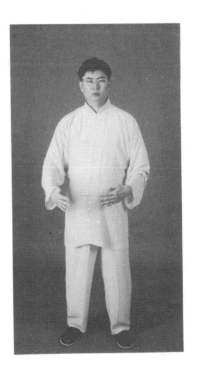

ACUTE CONDITION

NH: bladder area

FH: other side of the bladder, fingers pointing down a bit to help eliminate energy

Sound: 9-9, 9-9, jiu-jiu, jiu-jiu

Visualize: light dissipating from the bladder

CHRONIC CONDITION

STEP 1

NH: bottom of the bladder at the lower abdomen

FH: side of the bladder (3 minutes each side)

Sound: 9-9, 9-9, jiu-jiu. jiu-jiu

Visualize: light radiating from the bladder

STEP 2

NH: bladder

FH: lower abdomen

Sound: 9-9, 9-9, jiu-jiu, jiu-jiu

Visualize: light dissipating from the bladder

Notes: Constricted blood vessels in the wall of the bladder and the tract restrict blood flow, resulting in not enough energy in the tissues.

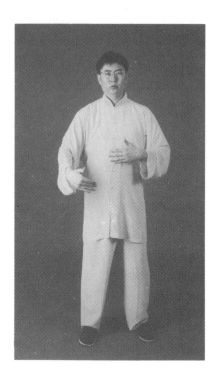

polyps or tumours in the urinary bladder

NH: middle finger points to polyps or tumours in the bladder

FH: lower abdomen (Lower Dan Tian)

Sound: 9-9, 9-9, *jiu-jiu, jiu-jiu*

Visualize: light dissipating from the bladder

enlarged or inflamed prostate

NH: middle finger points towards and shakes at the prostate

FH: lower abdomen (Lower Dan Tian)

Sound: 9-9, 9-9, jiu-jiu, jiu-jiu

Visualize: light dissipating in the prostate gland; imagine the prostate shrinking and getting smaller

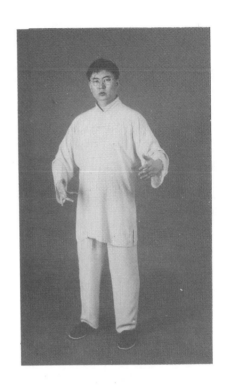

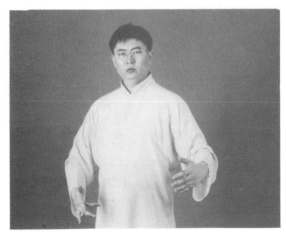

Conditions of the Lower Abdomen

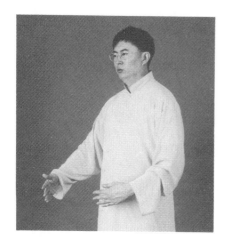

pain around the navel

NH: middle finger points towards the painful area

FH: another part of the abdomen

Sound: 9-9, 9-9, *jiu-jiu, jiu-jiu*

Visualize: light dissipating from the navel area

diarrhea

NH: lower abdomen (Lower Dan Tian)

FH: upper abdomen or the stomach area

Sound: 9-5, 9-5, *jiu-wu, jiu-wu*

Visualize: light flowing from the lower abdomen to the stomach

Notes: Diarrhea is caused by lack of cell activity in the digestive organs. If the condition persists, increase fluid intake to maintain electrolyte balance and to prevent dehydration of the body.

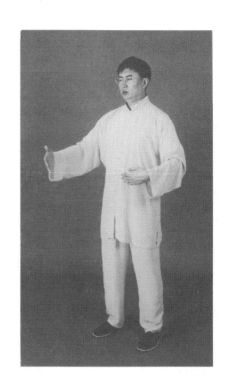

165

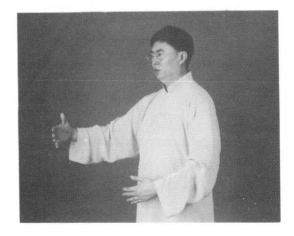

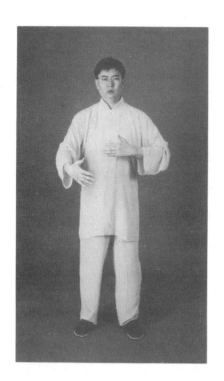

constipation

NH: upper abdomen

FH: lower abdomen (Lower Dan Tian)

Sound: 5-9, 5-9, *wu-jiu, wu-jiu*

Visualize: light flowing from the upper abdomen to the lower abdomen

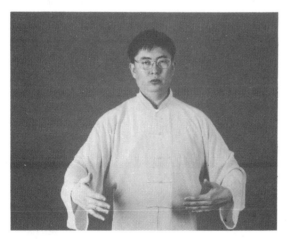

Feminine Conditions

uterine fibroids

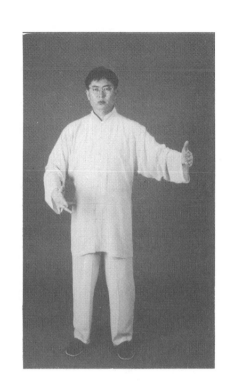

NH: middle finger points at the area of the fibroid(s) or tumour(s)

FH: side of the lower abdomen

Sound: 9-9, 9-9, *jiu-jiu, jiu-jiu*

Visualize: light dissipating from the uterus

Notes: Blood clots will form (a good sign) when the tumour begins dissipating. Continue with the treatment and the herbs prescribed. If uterine bleeding resumes (discharge changes from a brown colour to a red colour), stop the procedure and use the healing technique for **Heavy Periods** (see page 168).

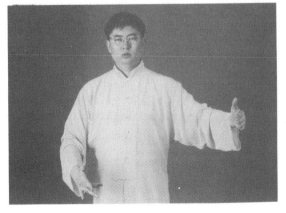

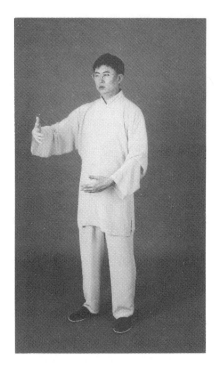

heavy periods (menorrhagia)

NH: uterus, palm facing slightly upwards

FH: upper abdomen, palm angled slightly downwards

Sound: 9-5, 9-5, *jiu-wu, jiu-wu*

Visualize: light flowing from the uterus to the upper abdomen

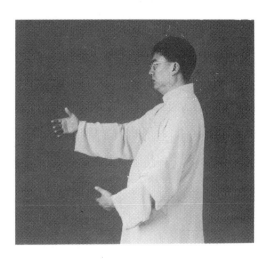

lumps in the breast, breast cysts and tumours

NH: middle finger points at the area of the cyst

FH: other breast

Sound: 3-3, 3-3, *san-san, san-san* or 2-2, 2-2, *ar-ar, ar-ar*

Visualize: light radiating from the cyst area

Notes: Alternate hands if there are cysts in both breasts.

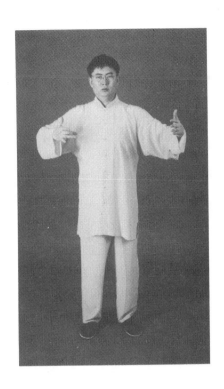

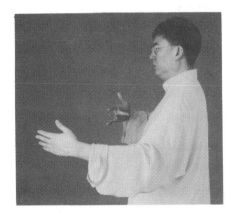

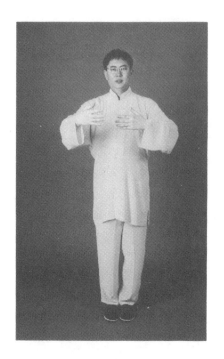

temperature imbalance in the body

NH: warm side of the body, at the chest or lung area

FH: the opposite side (the cold side) of the body

Sound: 2-2, 2-2, *ar-ar, ar-ar*

Visualize: light flowing from the warm part of the body to the cold part

Notes: Half of the body feels warm; the other half feels cold.

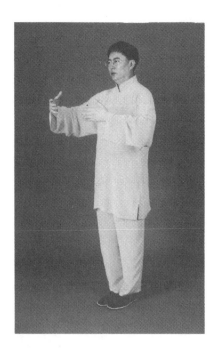

inflammation of the aorta (arteristis)

NH: center of the chest (Middle Dan Tian)

FH: fingers extended straight out and pointing away from the body

Sound: 2-2, 2-2, ar-ar, ar-ar

Visualize: light dissipating from the area of the heart

Notes: *Emergency situation! Get patient to hospital immediately! 3 minutes maximum*

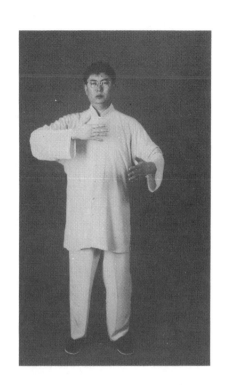

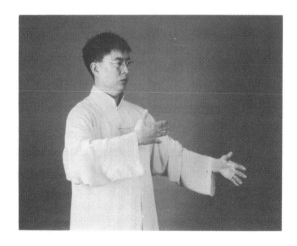

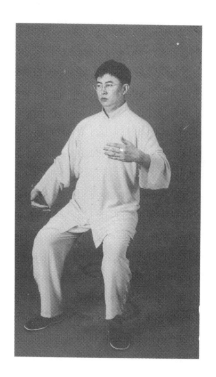

inflammation of the veins (phlebitis)

NH: 4 fingers point up the affected leg at the site of the inflamed veins

FH: right side of the heart, above the level of the nipple (the right auricle)

Sound: 11-2, 11-2, *shiyi-ar, shiyi-ar*

Visualize: light flowing from the affected veins to the right auricle of the heart

Notes: Seek acupuncture treatment for varicose veins. If there is a heavy feeling or swelling of the legs after standing or walking, work on improving circulation.

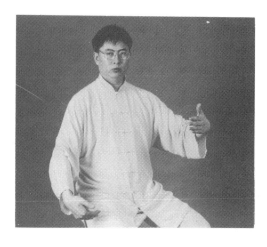

Cold Conditions

cold
(the lungs are clear)

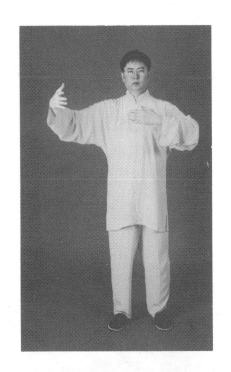

NH: center of chest, above nipple level

FH: above nipple level, facing the lungs

Sound: 3-5, 3-5, *san-wu, san-wu*

Visualize: light dissipating from chest

173

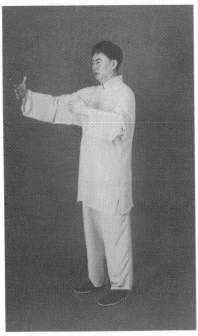

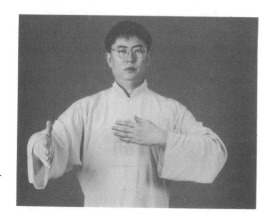

174

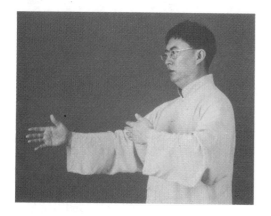

cold
(with high fever)

NH: center of chest, above the nipples

FH: extended straight out with the fingers pointing away from the body, above the level of the nipples

Sound: 3-5, 3-5, *san-wu, san-wu*

Visualize: light radiating and dissipating from the chest area

Notes: Do for 2 minutes only as energy is being directed away from the body with the extended *far hand.*

cold
(after blood loss)

NH: lower abdomen (Lower Dan Tian)

FH: lungs or the center of the chest, above the level of the nipples

Sound: 9-3, 9-3. *jiu-san, jiu-san*

Visualize: light flowing from the lower abdomen to the lungs

Notes: Use this procedure when the patient catches a cold after suffering blood loss from surgery or injury.

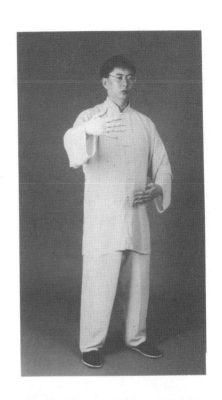

175

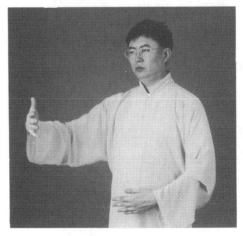

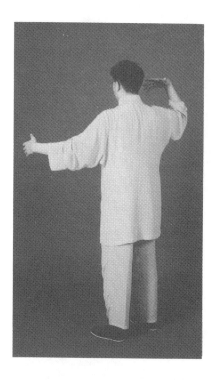

neck pain
(caused by wind)

NH: back of neck

FH: lower abdomen (Lower Dan Tian) or the lower back or the side of the body

Sound: 1-9, 1-9, *yi-jiu, yi-jiu*

Visualize: light flowing from neck to the lower abdomen (Lower Dan Tian)

Notes: Unprotected exposure to too much wind (natural energy) can accumulate as blocked energy in the body, causing pain and stiffness.

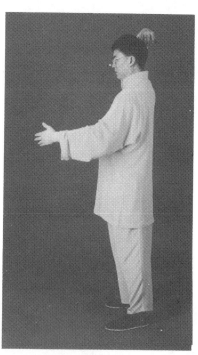

cervical bone spur

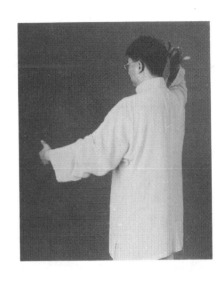

NH: middle finger points at the back of the neck at the affected area

FH: lower abdomen (Lower Dan Tian)

Sound: 1-9, 1-9, *yi-jiu, yi-jiu*

Visualize: light dissipating from the area of the spur

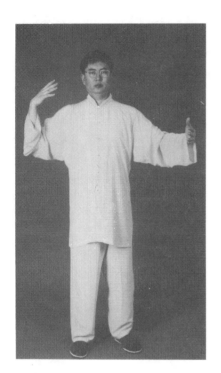

frozen shoulder

NH: palm faces the affected shoulder or the middle finger points to the affected shoulder

FH: chest area (Middle Dan Tian)

Sound: 11-5, 11-5, *shiyi-wu, shiyi-wu*

Visualize: light flowing from the affected shoulder to the chest

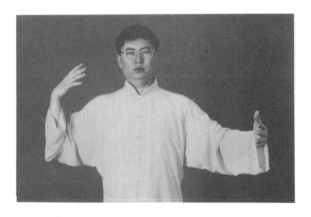

adhesions in shoulders (muscles and tendons stuck together)

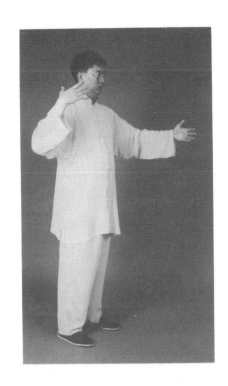

NH: over affected shoulder, shaking

FH: chest area (Middle Dan Tian)

Sound: 11-5, 11-5, *shiyi-wu, shiyi-wu*

Visualize: light dissipating in affected area

Notes: Patients with this condition feel as if the muscles and tendons in the shoulder area are stuck together.

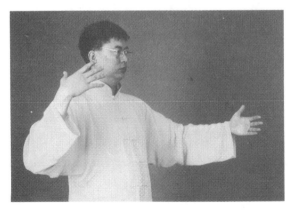

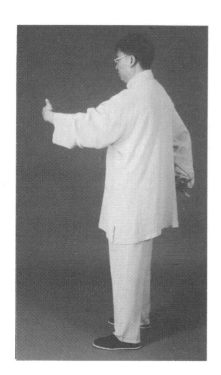

lower back problems, osteoarthritis, lumbar spine

NH: middle finger points upwards at the area affected

FH: ribs

Sound: 9-6, 9-6, *jiu-liu, jiu-liu*

Visualize: light dissipating from the affected area

slipped disc
(herniation of the lumbar disc)

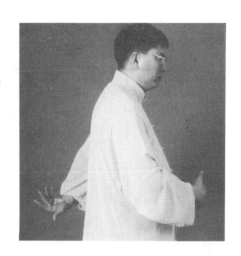

NH: lower abdomen (Lower Dan Tian)

FH: lower back, facing the area of the slipped disc

Sound: 9-9, 9-9, *jiu-jiu, jiu-jiu*

Visualize: light flowing from the lower abdomen (Lower Dan Tian) to the affected area

Notes: This condition is due to weak back energy (weak Du meridian), unless otherwise caused by trauma or sports injury. This problem seems to be more common with office workers than with manual labourers.

181

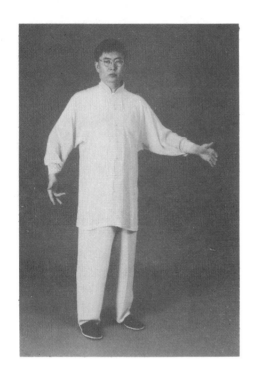

pain in the lower back and down the leg (sciatica)

NH: palm facing towards the affected area or use the middle finger to point to it

FH: other side of the body or the lower abdomen (Lower Dan Tian)

Sound: 11-9, 11-9, *shiyi-jiu, shiyi-jiu*

Visualize: light flowing from the affected area to the other side of the body or to the lower abdomen (Lower Dan Tian)

lower back pain

NH: facing the painful side of the back

FH: opposite side of the back

Sound: 9-9, 9-9, *jiu-jiu, jiu-jiu*

Visualize: light dissipating from the painful side of the back

Notes: Alternate the hands.

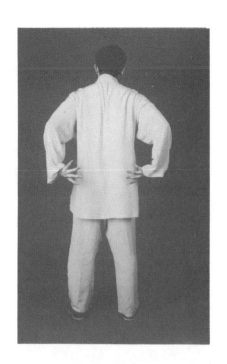

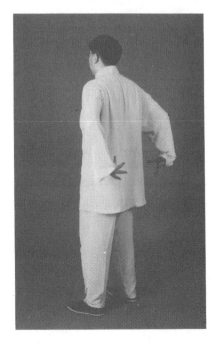

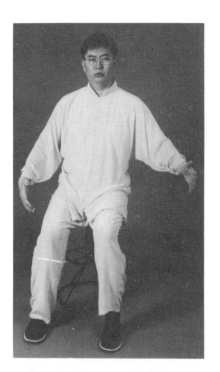

arthritic pain in the knee (osteoarthritis of the knee)

NH: affected knee

FH: other knee

Sound: 11, 11, *shiyi, shiyi*

Visualize: light dissipating in the area of the affected knee

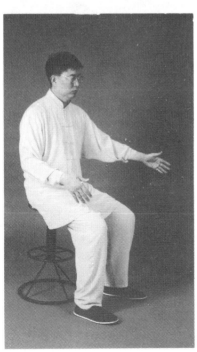

ankle pain

One Hand Method: point all 4 fingers at the affected area

Sound: 11, 11, *shiyi, shiyi*

Visualize: light dissipating from the ankle

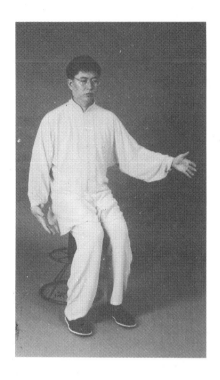

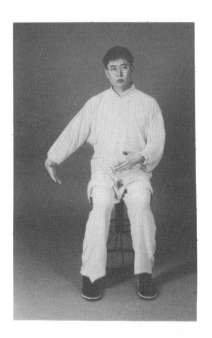

inflammation of the bone marrow (osteomyelitis)

NH: over the affected bone

FH: lower part of the affected area

Sound: 11, 11, *shiyi, shiyi*

Visualize: light flowing downwards from the affected area

Notes: This procedure directs energy downwards from the affected area, otherwise the infection can spread through the bone marrow.

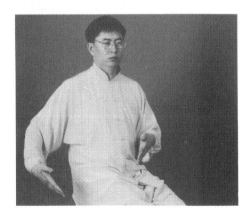

cavities in the bone marrow (osteomyelitic cavitation)

NH: lower abdomen (Lower Dan Tian)

FH: affected area

Sound: 9-9, 9-9, *jiu-jiu, jiu-jiu* or 9-11, *jiu-shiyi* (if treating a limb or an extremity of the body)

Visualize: light flowing from the Lower Dan Tian (lower abdomen) to the affected area

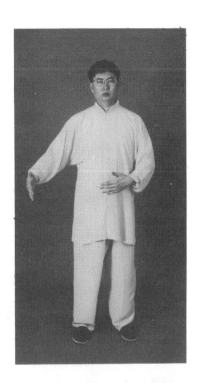

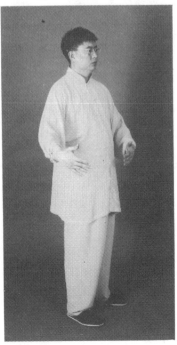

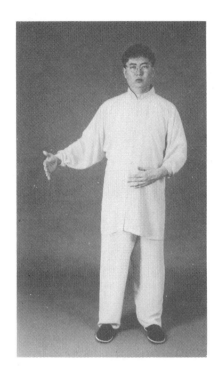

low bone density (osteoporosis)

NH: lower abdomen (Lower Dan Tian)

FH: affected area

Sound: 9-9, 9-9, *jiu-jiu, jiu-jiu*

Visualize: the bones and the whole skeleton glowing brightly with light and being strong, dense and full of energy

Notes: Think of the Snow Mountain Area strengthening the kidneys and building up energy there.

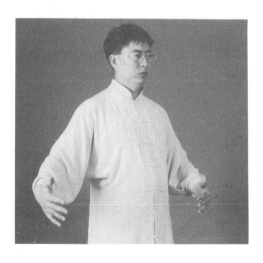

Skin Conditions

burn
(new)

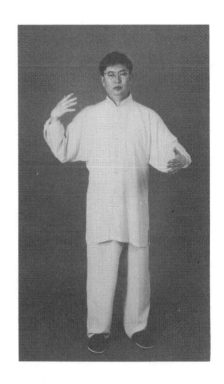

NH: area of the new burn

FH: lower abdomen (Lower Dan Tian)

Sound: X-9, X-9, *x-jiu, x-jiu*
(The healing number to use for the burn area depends on its location. Refer to Table 6 on page 83 for the healing numbers and the Mandarin pronunciations to use. Substitute the correct number in place of X and the correct pronunciation in place of *x* in the sound sequence shown above.)

Visualize: light flowing from the area of the burn to the Lower Dan Tian

Notes: New burns are areas where the tissues have too much energy. This method transfers the excess energy to the Lower Dan Tian, the body's storehouse of energy.

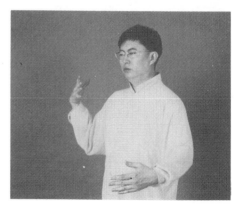

PHOTO EXAMPLE
(new burn on the face)

NH: face

FH: lower abdomen (Lower Dan Tian)

Sound: 1-9, 1-9, *yi-jiu, yi-jiu*

Visualize: light flowing from the facial burn to the Lower Dan Tian

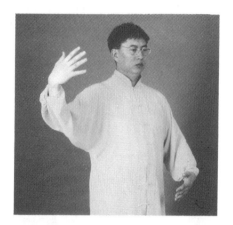

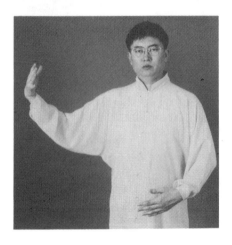

190

burn
(old)

NH: lower abdomen (Lower Dan Tian)

FH: burn area

Sound: 9-**X**, 9-X, *jiu-**x***, *jiu-**x***
(The healing number to use for the burn area depends on its location. Refer to Table 6 on page 83 for the healing numbers and the Mandarin pronunciations to use. Substitute the correct number in place of X and the correct pronunciation in place of **x** in the sound sequence shown above.)

Visualize: light flowing from the Lower Dan Tian to the burn area

Notes: Recovery of old burns is slow due to insufficient energy in the burn area. This method sends energy from the Lower Dan Tian to the area of the old burn.

PHOTO EXAMPLE
(old burn on the face)

NH: lower abdomen (Lower Dan Tian)

FH: face

Sound: 9-1, 9-1, *jiu-yi*, *jiu-yi*

Visualize: light flowing from the Lower Dan Tian to the burn area on the face

psoriasis
(of the head)

NH: upper side of the head

FH: other side of the head

Sound: 1-1, 1-1, *yi-yi, yi-yi*

Visualize: a knife cutting off the affected skin

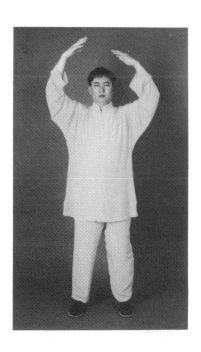

191

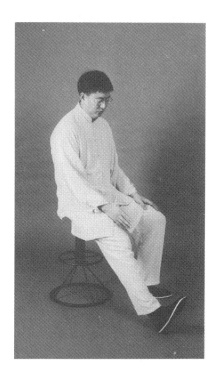

athlete's foot

One Hand Method: point all 4 fingers at the affected foot, fingers angled slightly upwards

Sound: 11, 11, *shiyi, shiyi*

Visualize: light dissipating from the affected area and the affected skin glowing bright with white light and being healthy

acne and facial blemishes

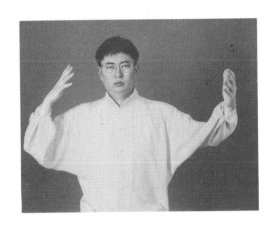

NH: middle finger points at the blemish or pimple

FH: any other part of the face

Sound: 1-1, 1-1, *yi-yi, yi-yi*

Visualize: light dissipating from the blemish or pimple

Notes: Alternate the hands if both sides of the face are affected.

193

Conclusion

Conclusion

This book has introduced the theories, principles and techniques of the new medical science of Zhi Neng medicine. Using the knowledge within, you can improve your own health and the health of your family and friends. For any health problem, refer to the book, study the pictures of the healing positions, and use the healing techniques. Reread the theories, principles and techniques, and think of how they apply to your situation.

The ultimate goal of Zhi Neng medicine is to teach the public and ordinary people to be responsible for their own health as much as possible. Also, Zhi Neng medicine complements the work of medical professionals, complementary health practitioners and other healers to offer the best health solution for the people in the world.

Practising Zhi Neng medicine will help you to develop and balance your energy for better health. Living by the principles of Zhi Neng medicine will develop your energy in body, mind and soul. The greatest gift is knowledge. Pass on what you have learned here to your family and friends.

This book is the first of a series on Zhi Neng medicine. The next book will discuss soul development, soul communication and soul healing.

Love one another. Touch with your heart. Help each other to heal. You are going to see a profound change in the world.

Welcome to the new world!

Thank you for supporting Zhi Neng medicine.

Thank you.

Appendix

Master Guo's Background

Master Zhi Chen Guo first started to learn the Chinese martial arts and Qi Gong at the age of ten. Now known as one of China's most famous Qi Gong masters, he has, after more than 30 years of practice, created Dong Yi Gong, the Zhi Neng medicine style of Qi Gong. A doctor of traditional Chinese medicine, he is also trained in and practices western medicine.

201

Guo's Sanitorium, a Qi Gong centre in Shijiazhuang, Tian Jing, China, was set up by Master Guo in 1986. After many years of study, he has combined elements of western medicine, traditional Chinese medicine, Qi Gong, and his own extraordinary functioning of the senses, to create the revolutionary, new health science of Zhi Neng medicine.

In 1992, before an audience of thousands, Master Guo introduced the principles, theories and techniques of Zhi Neng medicine to the public. He presented new principles, knowledge and concepts never before introduced, to develop and balance energy in the body, mind and soul.

He has also created a new discipline called *subconscious science*, which is more than Soul Study. The study of the soul includes soul development, soul communication, and soul healing. Thousands of Master Guo's Soul Study students have applied their knowledge of the soul with remarkable results in many fields, including health, physics, agriculture and business.

Another one of Master Guo's contributions to the world include finding the location of the *zhong gong* behind the portal vein. The *zhong gong* is the *life centre* and the basis of a person's life and its state is related to one's health. Your mind must be developed enough to be able to see it.

Zhi Neng medicine has spread rapidly in Asia and more recently in Canada as a result of Master Guo's revolutionary insights and theories.

Master Sha's Background

Master Zhi Gang Sha received his MD in Western Medicine from China's Xian Medical University in 1983. He is also a doctor of traditional Chinese medicine, skilled in the use of acupuncture, herbs and Chinese massage. He obtained his Masters' degree in Hospital Administration from the University of the Philippines (Manila) in 1988.

Since boyhood, he has practised many of the Eastern arts and studied under many masters and teachers of Buddhism, Taoism, Confucianism, I Ching, traditional Chinese medicine and acupuncture.

In 1978, Master Sha developed a unique acupuncture technique that has proven very effective for pain relief. Delivering results faster than traditional acupuncture methods, *Sha's Acupuncture* combines energy healing and involves only a few key acupuncture points. From 1986 to 1988, he taught Sha's Acupuncture, Qi Gong and Tai Chi at the World Health Organization's *Acupuncture and Qi Gong Training Centre* in Beijing. His students included hundreds of medical doctors from around the world.

Master Sha first encountered Zhi Neng medicine in 1989, and has since devoted his life to spreading its knowledge throughout the world. He became the first disciple and the adopted son of its founder, Master Zhi Chen Guo. He has lectured to hundreds of thousands internationally on the benefits of Zhi Neng medicine and on the pain-relieving aspects of Sha's Acupuncture. Invited by doctors, hospitals, health associations, support groups and many other organizations to give presentations on his healing work, he is also a popular keynote speaker at many conferences. He has been featured on television, on radio and in print media worldwide.

In 1995, Master Sha established the International Institute of Zhi Neng™ Medicine in Vancouver, BC, Canada.

The International Institute of Zhi Neng™ Medicine

Established in 1995, the International Institute of Zhi Neng™ Medicine is dedicated to spreading the knowledge, principles and techniques of Zhi Neng medicine to the public through its *healing* work and by *teaching*.

A wide range of illnesses are treated in the medical clinic operated by the Institute. Patients often experience remarkable results and make dramatic recoveries. Many experience true pain relief for the first time in years. Other services include *long-distance healing* and *soul consultations*.

203

Multi-level practitioner courses teach and qualify healers in *Zhi Neng medicine* and *Sha's Acupuncture Therapy. Dong Yi Gong* classes help students develop energy. *Self-healing* classes teach healing and energy balancing. *One-Week Intensive Healing* programs offer solutions for chronic pain. *Weight loss* clinics are ongoing. *Soul Study* offers revolutionary soul and spiritual development. As well, *feng shui* classes are being planned.

Books, video tapes and other material on Zhi Neng medicine, on healing and on how to improve the quality of life are available for purchase at the Institute. Topics include Soul Study, energy development, self-healing, weight loss, digestive problems, sinus problems, back pain and more.

The Institute often holds demonstrations and seminars for doctors, hospitals, support groups, the public and other interested parties, locally and internationally. For more information, please direct all inquiries to:

Zhi Gang Sha LLC
PO Box 470580
San Francisco, CA 94147-0580
Telephone: 1-888-339-6815 (Toll Free North America)
Website: www.drsha.com

Ailments and Conditions Helped with Zhi Neng Medicine

Zhi Neng medicine has been successful in treating a wide variety of medical conditions and many other health problems. The self-healing aspect of this *medicineless science* has proven particularly successful for conditions of chronic pain. You will see improved health and have a better quality of life when you practice Zhi Neng medicine self-healing techniques regularly and actively.

The following is a partial listing of some common ailments that Zhi Neng medicine has been successful in treating and in helping patients recover from.

Zhi Neng Medicine Helps Many Conditions

- Addictions (drugs, alcohol, etc.)
- Allergies
- Alzheimer's
- Arthritis
- Asthma
- Back Pain
- Bronchitis
- Bowel Disease
- Cancer, Cysts & Tumours
- Colds
- Deafness (nerve-related)
- Depression
- Diabetes
- Eye Problems
- Fatigue
- Feminine Problems
- Fibromyalgia
- Frozen Shoulder
- Heart Problems
- Impotence
- Incontinence
- Indigestion
- Injuries
- Insomnia
- Joint Problems
- Mental Disorders
- Migraines & Headaches
- Multiple Sclerosis
- Pain (acute and chronic)
- Parkinsonism
- Sciatica Nerve Problems
- Sports Injuries
- Stomach Problems
- Stroke-Related Paralysis
- Surgery Recovery
- Uterine Fibroids
- Weight Loss
- Whiplash

Post Treatment Care

Follow the guidelines below for *more effective recovery* from conditions you are having treated at the International Institute of Zhi Neng™ Medicine. If you are seeking relief from pain or have inflammation, swelling, cysts, unusual growths, follow these guidelines for as long as your condition persists.

205

Avoid All Foods in the Following Categories

- **SEAFOOD,** including salmon, tuna, trout, sushi, lobster, crab, shrimp, oysters, clams, anything that swims or lives in water, etc.
- **NUTS & SEEDS,** including almonds, peanuts, peanut butter, pumpkin seeds, sesame seeds, sunflower seeds, etc.
- **DRIED BEANS & LEGUMES,** including lentils, peas, chick peas, lima beans, baked beans, pea soup, homous, tofu, soy sauce, soy milk, etc. *Small amounts of legumes are permitted if you are following a vegan diet (totally vegetarian).*
- **CAFFEINE,** including chocolate, Cola drinks, coffee, tea (herbal teas OK)
- **DEEP FRIED FOODS,** including chips, fries, samosas, doughnuts
- **COLD FOODS & DRINKS**
- **ALCOHOL**

Recommended Diet

Your diet should consist of warm liquids, grains, vegetables and fruits.
If you do eat meat, eat small amounts of lean beef, chicken or pork.
Steam-cook food or use any other method that retains maximum nutrition.
If you have a skin condition, avoid all meats, dairy products and eggs.

Other Suggestions

KEEP WARM & DRY. Cover your head and neck in cold weather.

DO NOT IMMERSE IN WATER. (No swimming, hot tubs or baths; take a quick shower or use a wash cloth, instead.)

If you experience relief from your condition, do not keep mentally checking to see if it has returned. Instead, think of yourself as getting well. If the problem persists, get a few more treatments.

Practice energy development to build up your body's healing energy.

Institute Programs

Sha's Acupuncture
Certificate Program

Certificate courses are offered in the revolutionary new acupuncture method known as **Sha's Acupuncture** therapy.

Developed in 1978 by Zhi Gang Sha, CMD, CHHP, MHA, Sha's Acupuncture is a uniquely effective form of acupuncture, combining essential components of Western medicine, traditional Chinese medicine and Qi Gong. Hundreds of medical professionals from around the world have taken these courses, and added Sha's Acupuncture to their practices.

Designed for medical professionals, **Sha's Acupuncture Certificate Program** involves three levels of study. Level I offers basic theory and techniques for using Sha's Acupuncture in your own practice, and Levels II and III, advanced skills and techniques. Each level consists of two consecutive weekends of intense training. **There must be a one year practicum between each level.**

Sha's Acupuncture Is Unique!
- Only a **few key** acupuncture points used, **not** 300+ like traditional acupuncture
- Quick in/out needle application
- Releases chronic pain quickly
- Energy healing involved
- Faster patient recovery
- Easy to learn

Contact the International Institute of Zhi Neng™ Medicine for more information and the latest schedules for this program.

Sha's Energy Massage
Certificate Program

Sha's Energy Massage is a unique energy massage therapy combining essential components of western medicine, traditional Chinese medicine, Qi Gong and Soul Healing. Developed by Master Zhi Gang Sha after more than twenty years of clinical practice, Sha's Energy Massage is an effective solution for chronic pain.

Similar in principle to the acclaimed pain-relieving aspects of *Sha's Acupuncture therapy,* Sha's Energy Massage uses special massage techniques combined with energy healing. The practitioner's hands and fingers act on key acupressure points to relieve pain, release tension and stress. Regular practice promotes healthy energy and blood flow in patients and helps balance the physical, mental, emotional and spiritual aspects of their beings.

Sha's Energy Massage is open to members of the healing professions, alternative and complementary health practitioners, and the general public. Upon successful completion of the program, certified practitioners can offer Sha's Energy Massage as a healing service to the public.

Sha's Energy Massage Offers the Following Benefits!
- Effective pain relief and stress release
- Based on the same principles as *Sha's Acupuncture Therapy*
- Uses only a few key acupressure points
- Releases chronic pain quickly *without* needles
- Promotes the healthy flow of blood and energy
- Energy healing and soul healing involved

Contact the International Institute of Zhi Neng™ Medicine for more information and the latest schedules for this program.

Soul Study

Soul Development with Master Zhi Gang Sha

More and more, people are talking about the soul. The soul is inside your body. The soul can also leave your body, absorb natural energy and then come back to your body. When your life ends, the soul leaves your body. *Where does it go? How long will it be until its next life? Is your soul happy or not? How long does your soul want to stay in your body? Can you communicate with your soul? Do you know what your soul likes or doesn't like? What is food for the soul? Can you heal your body? How much healing power does your soul have?*

Everybody has a soul. Other highly evolved souls can visit your soul to enlighten you by their presence. *Will they stay or not? Do you want to know what special messages the universe has for you? How you can access them? How accurate is your message-reading ability?*

How do you communicate with your soul? What are the most effective and fastest techniques to develop your soul? The soul seeks to evolve by learning new things in every life. It is always searching for knowledge. *What happens if your soul and physical body are not in harmony? If you are sick, how can you call upon your soul and the higher souls to help you?*

Soul Study, a revolutionary seven-level course, addresses all these questions and teaches you how to communicate with your soul, increase your soul power and use your soul to heal your physical body.

The revolutionary techniques used for soul development, soul communication and soul healing were created by the founder of Zhi Neng Medicine, Master Zhi Chen Guo. Thousands of people in China and hundreds in Canada have successfully applied these techniques in every facet of their lives with remarkable results.

Knowledge of the soul and the soul world will help you in many ways. If your soul is highly developed, you can receive messages from the universe. You will know about past lives and events, future events and even your future lives. Start creating harmony within your body, mind and soul. Receive guidance and direction on every thing that you do.

Soul Study opens up new dimensions. Start interacting beyond the physical world. Know that you have saints and guides with you and that you are not alone. Start attending to matters on the spiritual plane. Respect the soul world.

Take up *Soul Study* if your soul is important to you.

Master Sha's
5 Day Intensive Healing Program
Solutions for Chronic Pain

*I*n my 20 years of medical experience in China, the Philippines, Hong Kong, Taiwan, the USA and Canada, I find that many people with chronic pain suffer for years, even decades, with little or no improvement. I have always thought, *"There must be a solution! They suffer too much. They have to know how to heal themselves. They have to learn scientific, effective self-healing techniques to help themselves."*

After years of successfully treating chronic pain sufferers of many ailments, I have developed a **Five Day Intensive Healing Program** for people who suffer from chronic pain.

Zhi Neng Medicine views all chronic pain as one of two types. One is *excess energy* or blocked energy and the other is *deficient energy* in specific parts of the body. Participants of the **Five Day Intensive Healing Program** receive *Sha's Acupuncture Therapy, Chinese herbs* (optional), and *Zhi Neng medicine self-healing* and *group-healing* classes. These all combine to help them remove energy blockages, develop and balance their energy and restore their health much faster. These are my solutions for chronic pain.

Not every condition of chronic pain can be completely relieved in five days. However, within this time, many people suffering from chronic pain will experience much relief. The Zhi Neng medicine *self-healing* and *energy development* techniques they learn can be practiced at home. This is where people can start taking care of their own health. The program works with patients, family members, friends, family doctors and complementary health practitioners to bring forth the best solution yet for sufferers of chronic pain.

Thank you very much for your participation and support.

Best wishes to every patient. Restore your health as soon as possible.

Thank you.

Testimonials and Comments

Doctors' Comments

- "<u>I (am) impressed</u> with the simplicity and effectiveness of his approaches, the definite and often remarkable benefit patients experience...."
  Nelie C. Johnson, MD, Maple Ridge, BC

- "<u>I am a medical oncologist</u> (and) am quite impressed with (Sha's) expertise in applying acupuncture to various patients with cancer who have failed standard type therapy available on this continent."
  SM Reingold, MD, MSc, FRCP(C), Brampton, Ontario

- "<u>It is comforting</u> to at last have found a treatment that works for many conditions, which unfortunately are mostly left unresolved after using traditional western medicine treatments and intervention alone."
  Donald W. Stewart, MD, Vancouver, BC

- "<u>Sha's Acupuncture Therapy</u> concentrates energy and directs it through the needle, creating an explosive force that opens up the areas of accumulated energy to balance them."
  Wen-Hsiung Chen, Ph.D., Professor (Physics), Taiwan

- "<u>Dr. Sha (treats)</u> many difficult and chronic patients with very good results both in China and in the Philippines, and he is fully appreciated by the patients."
  WP Chang, MD, MPH, World Health Organization (Office of the Western Pacific)

MD WRITES IN:
Patients Improved with Zhi Neng Medicine

It is with great pleasure that I introduce to you Dr. (Master) Zhi Gang Sha who is a very uniquely qualified health practitioner. Dr. Sha has several outstanding credentials, having received his M.D. Degree in Western Medicine from China's Xian Medical College in 1983, and also a Diploma in traditional Chinese medicine, an expert in acupuncture and a master of Qi Gong.

Dr. Sha has developed a more simplified form of acupuncture essentially using less than twenty points for treating most medical conditions. This is a great advantage compared to the traditional Chinese acupuncture system which uses hundreds of points on the meridians. Dr. Sha has also been an instructor of Qi Gong and acupuncture at the World Health Organization Acupuncture Training Center in Beijing. Master Sha instructed doctors from all around the world.

Synthesizing all of the above disciplines and combining them has produced a revolutionary new health science now called Zhi Neng Medicine.

I have received treatments of Zhi Neng Medicine myself from Dr. Sha and so have several of my patients. I certainly can say that I myself am feeling much more energetic and all of the patients are also improved. It is comforting to at last have found a treatment that works for many conditions which unfortunately are mostly left unresolved after using traditional western medicine treatments and interventions alone.

We are most fortunate in Vancouver that Dr. Sha has come and that he is very willing to share his knowledge and methods of treatment. The treatments are very simple and practical and can be learned by most individuals as self healing techniques for health improvement and maintenance.

Thank you Master Sha for helping us all and for the joy and dedication with which you carry out your seemingly never ending work.

Donald W. Stewart, M.D.
Family Practice in Preventive Medicine
Vancouver, BC
February 28, 1996

BACK PAIN:

Thanks for Giving Me Back My Life!

For thirteen years I suffered with severe and often disabling back pain caused by bone deformities in my spine and subsequent nerve damage.

Some days I was not able to stand or walk; I had weakness and numbness in my feet. I underwent three surgeries and more than forty caudal infusions in the hope of eliminating the pain. Sleep was often elusive, and during my bad spells, I would sleep only two to three hours per night for days on end. I attended two pain clinics and explored alternative therapies, always searching for the hope that my future would not entail endless days of pain. In the Spring of '95 my feelings of hopelessness changed to hopefulness.

My husband happened to see an interview on television where Dr. Sha demonstrated his revolutionary form of acupuncture. On this program, Dr. Sha relieved a man of his chronic migraine headache in a matter of seconds. As well, there were patients who attested to Dr. Sha's success in reversing their cancers. My husband was impressed and said to me, "*This is the man you need to see!*"

At first when I arrived in Toronto, I was hopeful but skeptical that something so simple could really help my case. After the first treatment I knew that my pain would be eliminated, and I decided to take other workshops with Dr. Sha. I learned how to develop and balance the energy of my body, as well as how to effect self-healing for chronic pain so that I would be able to maintain improved health for myself.

Today I am able to lead a normal life and my future promises to be exciting. On days when I do more than my teenagers can tolerate, I sometimes feel the old pain returning, but now I have the skills to manifest self-healing and I am able to sleep peacefully at night.

I give heartfelt thanks to Dr. Sha and Zhi Neng Medicine for giving me back my life! Thank You.

Brigida Milne, Hope, BC
September 1996

ARTHRITIS:

Bone Fusion Reversing

I had my first arthritic experience at age 15. That was for two days. I could hardly move. Felt like an old man. Was very scared. It went away completely. It seemed to anyway.

When I was 19, both of my knees were swollen like softballs. That lasted for two to three months. Four months later it came back. That's when it started coming back every fall and winter. In the spring it would subside, it completely left me. Medically they called it *in remission.* But it would come back in the fall. Till I was 21. After the second year I had a major crisis. Then it was with me all year permanently for the last eight years.

I also had colitis from taking nonsteroidal anti-inflammatory (NSA) drugs. The colitis stayed with me for one to two years. After two years of colitis I stopped all drugs.

I was on seven types of drugs. Drugs for arthritis to stop the inflammation, drugs for the colon, drugs for protecting the stomach against ulcers. My colon was open and bleeding all the time. They wanted to remove my colon with an operation. I had blood transfusions for the colon. I came close to death three to four times.

I've been in a wheelchair for three years; before that I was bedridden for one to three years, off and on. The cartilage in my hips were worn down to the point where it was bone-on-bone. I've had both hips replaced with ball and socket joints. My hips were replaced one and a half years ago; I'm learning to walk again.

I've been coming for two weeks for treatment with Master Sha. My sacrum was fused. Since coming to see Master Sha, it has opened up. Master Sha has reversed the bone fusion. My spine was curved, it is now straight. My energy level is much higher. I feel very inspired because Master Sha has taught me how to heal myself with *Dong Yi Gong.*

My *Five Day Healing* class is teaching me much about the laws of healing and the universe. The two treatments per day of acupuncture that go along with the classes are beneficial and I feel that my body and being are going through transformations. I feel and know that I am becoming renewed and I know that I will completely recover from all disease through Master Sha's program of healing and group support.

(I AM HEALTH ABSOLUTE) Troy Davids, Vancouver, BC
February 8, 1996

213

DEAFNESS:
TV Station Owner Hears with Dud Ear

"Henry Lum is one of the many Chinese-Canadians who take advantage of both eastern and western medicine. For some things, like flus and colds, he'll go to Vancouver's Chinatown for herbs. For others, he'll consult his doctor.

Already a convert to *tai chi* for about 25 years, Lum, 59, who owns Ambleside TV in West Vancouver, went to learn more about *qi gong* from a Sha lecture. Once there, his wife nudged him forward to ask Sha to treat his right ear, which had been pretty much a dud for four years. Although his doctor had urged Lum to see a specialist, Lum had a functioning left ear, so he never bothered. He got by and if he couldn't hear his wife because he was lying down on his left ear, well, so be it, he had thought.

Besides, Zhi Neng involved acupuncture, which involved needles, which terrified him. "She pushed me out there," he says, explaining how he ended up asking Sha to look at his ear.

Sha inserted a few of those needles into him and when he removed therm, he picked up the phone and told Lum to call someone. He called his son's home and clearly heard his daughter-in-law's voice with his dud ear.

That was last March and five months later, he is sound of hearing."

Excerpt from *The Chinese Energizer,* an article on Dr. Sha in the *For Your Information* section, the VANCOUVER SUN, July 18, 1994

BACK PAIN:
My Revived Energy Level is Incredible

I am so very grateful to you Master Sha for the change your treatments and classes have made in my life. The acupuncture treatments for my 30 year back pain - 2 degenerating discs - has allowed me to be relatively pain free with a great deal more mobility.

What I love the most is the vitality I get from the Qi Gong Classes and following a daily ritual of 30 minutes of Qi Gong from the tapes. My revived energy level is incredible. I also use the 3396815 for relieving stress - when I'm upset over something - I just keep repeating until I am calm - even use it when I am driving.

Words alone cannot convey my appreciation, my heart is very grateful. Thank you.

Vida Crawford, Vancouver, BC
January 24, 1996

STROKE:

Making Cakes & Pies After 5 Treatments

My mother had a mild stroke, which, added to the continued symptoms from a car accident one year prior, left her with dizziness; blackouts; choking from inability to swallow; loss of feelings in her face, fingers, and feet; slurring of speech; anxiety attacks, urinary incontinence, and more. My mother, Alice, went from a strong spirited, hard-working soul to someone who tearfully wondered if she would make it to Christmas.

Within her first treatment with Master Sha, my mother's speech was noticeably restored, her swallowing returned to normal, she had no more urinary incontinence, and she once again had hope.

215

Just last week, after five treatments, she made a 15 pound carrot cake, three large lemon pies and lots of other goodies for 60 people at Saturday's Christmas Soccer party. I wonder if those kids will ever know how significant this gesture was.

Lorna J. Hancock, Executive Director, Health Action Network Society (HANS), Burnaby, BC
December 20, 1995

BRAIN SURGERY:

I Think Dr. Sha Put A Can of Oil in the Joints

I had brain surgery three years previous and after all the drugs, gained 30 pounds in weight. (I) did not have vertical (sense) of gravity. (I also had) a dead pelvic area.

With training, I have beaten all the odds for someone (who should) be in a box. I have learned to walk without my wheelchair and parked my walker. (I am) using no equipment and now feel wonderful. The perfectionist (that) I am is not agreeable that I am walking crooked.

Master Sha has worked on me many times and I am improving a lot, thank goodness. The crooked road is becoming straighter. It's been a long three years and my life is being put back together.

Another year just around the corner and hopefully (I) will be (walking) straight. I think Dr. Sha put a can of oil in the joints.

Jean Amadatsu, Vancouver, BC
December 29, 1995

CANCER:

Pancreatic Cancer Shrinks By More Than Half

I am writing to you (Dr. Sha) on behalf of my mother, Mrs. Binh Huynh Phung, to thank you for your extraordinary care of her pancreatic problem. In May 1994, she had obvious jaundice, lost her desire for food and lost weight. You believed she had a pancreatic problem and advised her to go through an emergency physical examination.

The examination was done at the Sunnybrook Health Centre. A minor operation was performed to correct the blockage in her pancreas. On the exam, the medical staff informed us that she had cancer, that their hands were tied and nothing could be done to restore her good health. She only had a few months to live. They encouraged her to undergo traditional Chinese herbal intensive therapy provided by you. From then on, she has continued with your therapy.

In the first few months, you had been seeing her seven days a week. Your treatment consisted of acupuncture, ancient Chinese *Qi Gong,* subconscious mind power and traditional Chinese herbal therapy. She has had a good appetite and has been feeling exceptionally well. The size of the cancer was initially 4.7 cm. and is now only 2.3 cm. She has been gaining weight.

My mother claims she is on her way to a good recovery. Now, she only needs to see you three times a week. Thank you for your remarkable therapy that has had no side effects but beneficial results.

Susie Chan, Don Mills, ON
September 8, 1995

SOUL'S QUEST:
Studying with a Rare Teacher

My soul's quest has lead me to Vancouver where I have the privilege of studying with a truly rare and exceptional teacher, Master Sha Zhi Gang.

It is with great joy and exhilaration that I embark on this journey of spiritual quest with very powerful lessons that are changing the way I experience my life. Throughout his lectures Master Sha brings his unique clarity and synthesis of spiritual knowledge and practical wisdom to the topic.

217

Master Sha's work has made a tremendous impact in my life and the lives of other practitioners. I have been most deeply affected by his teachings as well as his dynamic approach to healing. Through his loving presence he uplifts and empowers our evolution and leads us to wholeness, fulfilment and spiritual growth. His knowledge is exemplary, his healings evident, his communications truthful as he focuses on developing clarity, humility, forgiveness and love.

I am eternally grateful and appreciative. I thank you, my cherished Teacher and I look forward to our continued service together with devotion, commitment and service.

Bozena Sacha, Toronto, ON
January 25, 1996

SPORTS INJURY:
Family Doctor Impressed with the Healing Progress

When I came to you on the 10th of January I had no idea what I was in for. All I knew was that my ankle was very badly sprained and my doctor told me I would not be healed properly for at least six to seven months.

I damaged the tendons on both sides of my ankle playing a sport (volleyball) I like very much. I came to Master Sha less than twenty four hours after the accident and I am glad I did. The compassion and willingness of the students to learn about "sports" injuries was my first indication that maybe I could be helped.

After three sessions with Master Sha, my family doctor was impressed with the healing progress I was making. After the fourth session with Master Sha I am walking, cautiously, but never the less walking with little or no pain. This progress was made in less than seven days.

Terry W. Bunke, Vancouver, BC
January 18, 1996

Index

For individual ailments, refer to the CONTENTS and the Healing Methods for Over 100 Common Ailments (pages 96 - 193)

221

Notes

Notes

Notes